CONTENTS

ANATOMY FOR

HIP OPENERS

AND

FORWARD BENDS

RAY LONG, MD, FRCSC

bandha yoga publications

Published by Bandha Yoga Publications
Plattsburgh, NY
www.bandhayoga.com

Distributed by Greenleaf Book Group LLC

For ordering information and bulk purchases, contact Bandha Yoga Publications.
info@bandhayoga.com
Phone: 518.578.3720

Design and composition by Greenleaf Book Group LLC
Cover design by Greenleaf Book Group LLC
Front and back cover illustrations by Kurt Long, BFA   www.kurtlong.net
Computer Graphics Technical Director: Chris Macivor
Sanskrit calligraphy and border painting: Stewart Thomas   www.palmstone.com
Editor: Eryn Kirkwood, MA, RYT   www.barrhavenyoga.com

ISBN 13: 978-1-60743-942-4

Part of the Tree Neutral™ program, which offsets the number of trees consumed in the production and printing of this book by taking proactive steps, such as planting trees in direct proportion to the number of trees used: www.treeneutral.com

Printed in Canada on acid-free paper

10 11 12 13 14 15   10 9 8 7 6 5 4 3 2 1

First Edition

INTRODUCTION

AS THE CHINESE PROVERB STATES, WHEN YOU CANNOT REACH AN IMPORTANT GOAL, keep the goal but change your strategy. Yoga poses, like goals, can sometimes be difficult to achieve. What are your options when you cannot attain a posture? You can give up on progressing in the pose or you can change your approach to attain it. Changing strategies requires resourcefulness. Draw on this to break through blockages and safely attain the asanas. The Mat Companion series provides you with these resources in the form of scientific techniques.

Suppose you have tried all of the conventional means to bring your thighs to the floor in Baddha Konasana (Bound Angle Pose). You've tried pressing the knees down or placed weights on the legs and still you haven't progressed. Continued attempts will likely yield little in the way of results. So you decide to change your strategy. You can apply facilitated stretching to lengthen the muscles that are preventing you from going deeper into the pose. In the process, not only will you be able to bring the thighs closer to the floor, but you will also stimulate the nerve receptors in the pelvic region. This will illuminate the first and second chakras and aid to open energetic blockages. In addition, practicing in this way brings a better understanding of the asymmetries in your body. This understanding will carry over into other poses, expanding your overall yoga experience.

Perhaps you have lower back strain in a forward bend. The temptation might be to give up on the pose. Instead, try engaging the abdominals to create reciprocal inhibition of the stretching back muscles. Contracting the abdominals also elicits the abdominal "air bag" effect and supports the lumbar spine. This change in strategy is simple to apply and often works. These are examples of how to combine your knowledge of Western science with the wisdom of Hatha Yoga.

In many ways, practicing yoga is like the work of a native rainmaker who performs a ceremony to release atmospheric tension. Yoga releases physical and spiritual tension. Be resourceful and strategic as you make rain, both as a practitioner and as a teacher.

HOW TO USE THIS BOOK

Practicing yoga is like passing through a series of doors, with each door revealing new possibilities in the poses. The key to unlocking the first door is understanding the joint positions. This understanding can be used to identify the muscles that create the form of the pose and those that stretch. The key to positioning the joints is engaging the correct muscles. This begins with the prime movers. Engage the prime movers and the bones will align. The key to deepening the asanas is using your understanding of physiology to lengthen the muscles that stretch in the pose. Focus on these keys and the postures will automatically fall into place and manifest the beneficial effects of yoga. These include improved flexibility, heightened awareness, a sense of well-being, and deep relaxation.

The Mat Companion series is a set of modular books. Each book focuses on a specific pose category and contains the following:

- **The Key Concepts:** a description of biomechanical and physiological principles with applications for specific poses.
- **The Bandha Yoga Codex:** a simple five-step process that can be used to improve your flexibility, strength, and precision in the asanas.
- **The Pose Section:** a detailed description of the individual postures.
- **Movement Index:** explanations of body movement and tables listing the muscles associated with each movement.
- **Anatomy Index:** a visual listing of bones, ligaments, and muscles (showing the origins, insertions, and actions of each).
- **Glossary of Terms**
- **Sanskrit Pronunciation and Pose Index**
- **English Pose Index**

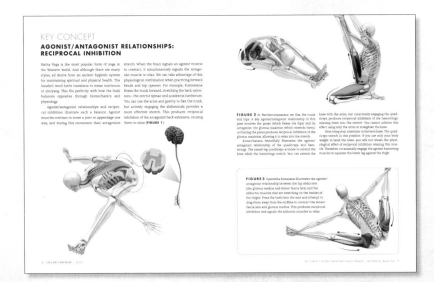

FIGURE 1 The Key Concepts show you how to apply biomechanics and physiology to your poses. Read this section first and return here often to refresh your knowledge.

FIGURE 2 The opening page for each pose illustrates the basic joint actions and positions of the body for that particular asana. Sanskrit and English names are provided for each posture. Use this page to assist you in learning the basic form of the pose and other concise details.

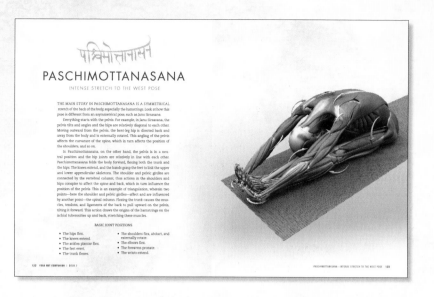

FIGURE 3 Use the preparatory section as a guide for how to enter the pose. If you are new to yoga or feel a bit stiff, use one of these modifications for your practice. In general, the preparatory poses affect the same muscle groups as the final asana. You will benefit from the pose no matter which variation you practice.

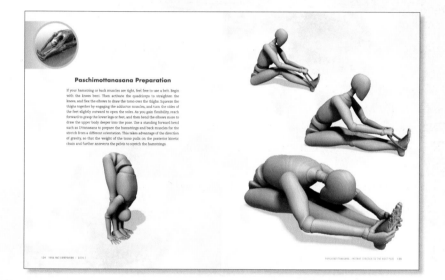

FIGURE 4 Each pose comes with a series of steps for engaging the muscles that position the joints, concluding with a summary of the muscles that stretch. Muscles that contract are colored different shades of blue (with the prime movers deep blue), and those that stretch are red. Use the pose section to master the anatomy of any given asana.

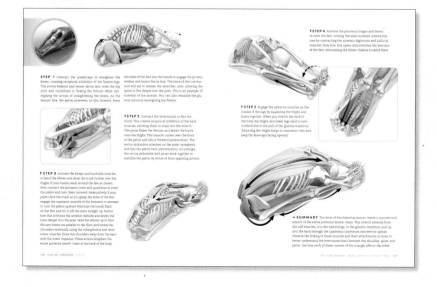

DESIGN STRATEGIES FOR YOGA PRACTICE

Visual artists often use identifiable techniques to draw their viewers' attention to a subject or to bring it into focus. **Grouping, repetition,** and **continuity** are three such examples. These same three techniques can be applied to your yoga practice. To use grouping, you can combine similar poses as we have done in the Mat Companion series. To apply repetition, stimulate a muscle group such as the psoas and its synergists several times during one session to bring it under conscious control. Continuity can be created by combining asanas so that they flow synergistically one into another. For maximum effect, simultaneously apply all three techniques—grouping, repetition, and continuity. In this way, the benefits of your practice will become greater than the sum of its parts.

I use this technique in the Psoas Awakening Series. In this practice, you combine the standing poses in a continuous series while repeatedly stimulating the psoas. This brings the muscle, which is generally difficult to access, into conscious awareness. Once the psoas has awakened, it will automatically engage whenever it can assist in achieving other yoga poses. Use grouping, repetition, and continuity when designing your practice and when teaching.

At the other end of the spectrum is a technique that artists use to introduce an element of chance and randomness into their work. Using this tool, a designer will take a pair of scissors to a literary work, cut it into pieces, and then randomly recombine it. The outcome is often remarkable. This parallels other methods of divination, such as the ancient Chinese book of wisdom, the I Ching. With the I Ching, one asks a question and then tosses coins in a seemingly random fashion. The pattern of the coins is then correlated with a hexagram that speaks to the question, often in profound ways. These methods strategically remove the intellect from the equation and provide access to the unconscious mind and the unseen world.

You can use this same technique in yoga. It is especially beneficial if you regularly follow a prescribed series of poses. Once a month, draw five asanas out of a hat. Carefully examine each one to understand its components. Consider how they are interrelated. Then combine the postures into a practice. This will profoundly impact your understanding of all the asanas. You might also come upon some great new sequences. Use the Mat Companion series to assist in your analysis of the poses.

KEY CONCEPTS

KEY CONCEPT

AGONIST/ANTAGONIST RELATIONSHIPS: RECIPROCAL INHIBITION

Hatha Yoga is the most popular form of yoga in the Western world. And although there are many styles, all derive from an ancient hygienic system for maintaining spiritual and physical health. The Sanskrit word *hatha* translates to mean sun/moon or yin/yang. This fits perfectly with how the body balances opposites through biomechanics and physiology.

Agonist/antagonist relationships and reciprocal inhibition illustrate such a balance. Agonist muscles contract to move a joint or appendage one way, and during this movement their antagonists stretch. When the brain signals an agonist muscle to contract, it simultaneously signals the antagonist muscle to relax. We can take advantage of this physiological combination when practicing forward bends and hip openers. For example, Kurmasana flexes the trunk forward, stretching the back extensors—the erector spinae and quadratus lumborum. You can use the arms and gravity to flex the trunk, but actively engaging the abdominals provides a more effective stretch. This produces reciprocal inhibition of the antagonist back extensors, causing them to relax. **FIGURE 1▼**

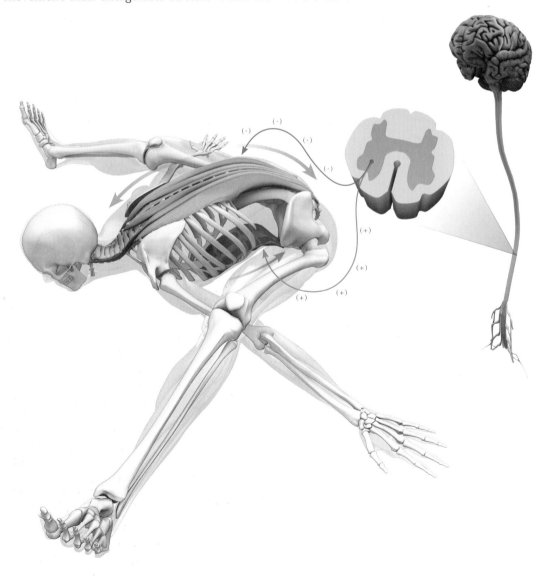

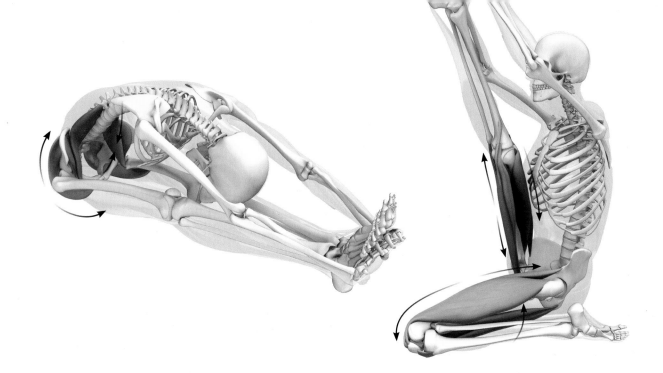

FIGURE 2 In Paschimottanasana we flex the trunk and hips. A key agonist/antagonist relationship in this pose involves the psoas (which flexes the hips) and its antagonist, the gluteus maximus (which extends them). Activating the psoas produces reciprocal inhibition of the gluteus maximus, allowing it to relax into the stretch.

Krounchasana beautifully illustrates the agonist/antagonist relationship of the quadriceps and hamstrings. The raised-leg quadriceps activate to extend the knee while the hamstrings stretch. You can extend the knee with the arms, but consciously engaging the quadriceps produces reciprocal inhibition of the hamstrings, relaxing them into the stretch. You cannot achieve this effect using only the arms to straighten the knee.

Now, bring your attention to the bent knee. The quadriceps stretch in this position. If you use only your body weight to bend the knee, you will not obtain the physiological effect of reciprocal inhibition relaxing this muscle. Therefore, occasionally engage the agonist hamstring muscles to squeeze the lower leg against the thigh.

FIGURE 3 Upavistha Konasana illustrates the agonist/antagonist relationship between the hip abductors (the gluteus medius and tensor fascia lata) and the adductor muscles that are stretching on the insides of the thighs. Press the heels into the mat and attempt to drag them away from the midline to contract the tensor fascia lata and gluteus medius. This produces reciprocal inhibition and signals the adductor muscles to relax.

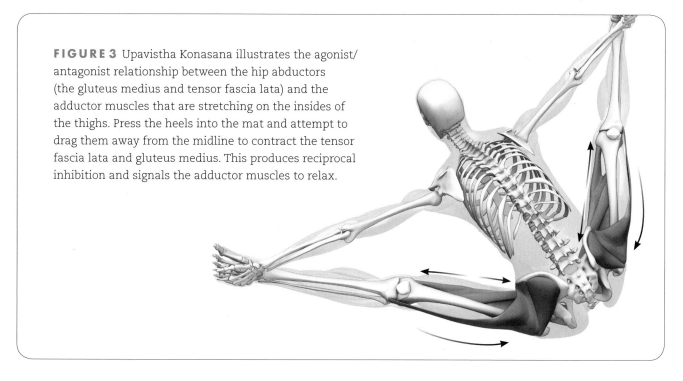

KEY CONCEPT
KEY MUSCLE ISOLATIONS

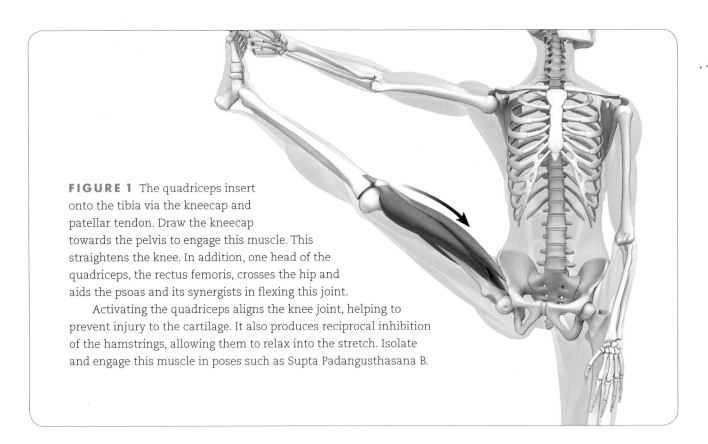

FIGURE 1 The quadriceps insert onto the tibia via the kneecap and patellar tendon. Draw the kneecap towards the pelvis to engage this muscle. This straightens the knee. In addition, one head of the quadriceps, the rectus femoris, crosses the hip and aids the psoas and its synergists in flexing this joint.

Activating the quadriceps aligns the knee joint, helping to prevent injury to the cartilage. It also produces reciprocal inhibition of the hamstrings, allowing them to relax into the stretch. Isolate and engage this muscle in poses such as Supta Padangusthasana B.

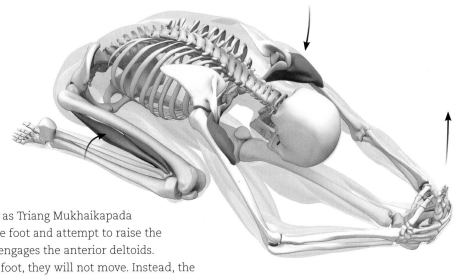

FIGURE 2 In forward bends such as Triang Mukhaikapada Paschimottanasana, firmly grasp the foot and attempt to raise the arms upwards toward the sky. This engages the anterior deltoids. Because the hands are gripping the foot, they will not move. Instead, the contracting deltoids draw the trunk deeper into the forward fold. At the same time, squeeze the bent-leg calf against the thigh. This activates the hamstrings, helping to maintain alignment of the knee joint.

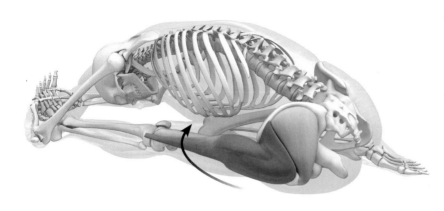

FIGURE 3 Press the heel of the straight-leg foot into the mat and attempt to drag it to the side in Triang Mukhaikapada Paschimottanasana; that is, attempt to abduct the leg. This engages the tensor fascia lata and gluteus medius, which in addition to being abductors of the thigh, are internal rotators of the hip. The foot remains fixed on the mat, so the force of the contraction shifts the body weight back toward the bent-knee side. This force is also transmuted to internal rotation of the thigh. Use this cue to bring the kneecap back to a neutral position from external rotation.

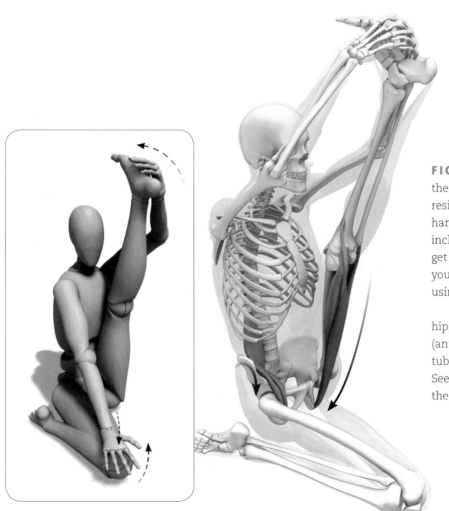

FIGURE 4 In Krounchasana, press the palm onto the bent knee and then resist as you try to lift the leg into the hand. This activates the hip flexors, including the psoas muscle. Once you get a feeling for engaging the psoas, you will be able to contract it without using the hand for resistance.

Note that, in addition to flexing the hip, the psoas also tilts the pelvis forward (anteversion). This draws the ischial tuberosities back away from the knee. See how this cue can be used to augment the stretch of the straight-leg hamstrings.

KEY CONCEPT
KEY CO-ACTIVATIONS

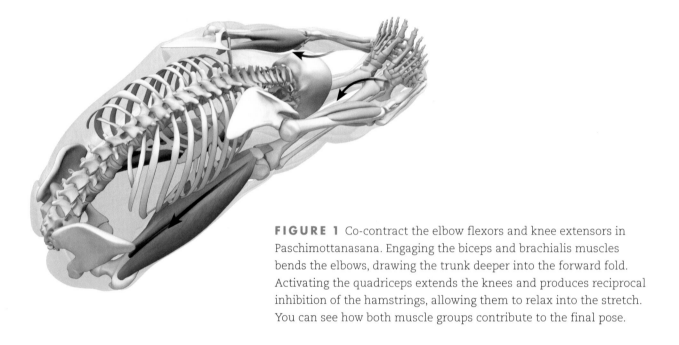

FIGURE 1 Co-contract the elbow flexors and knee extensors in Paschimottanasana. Engaging the biceps and brachialis muscles bends the elbows, drawing the trunk deeper into the forward fold. Activating the quadriceps extends the knees and produces reciprocal inhibition of the hamstrings, allowing them to relax into the stretch. You can see how both muscle groups contribute to the final pose.

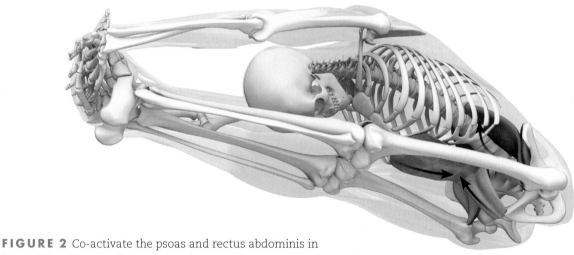

FIGURE 2 Co-activate the psoas and rectus abdominis in forward bends. A cue for engaging the psoas is to squeeze the torso against the thighs. Contracting these muscles together flexes both the trunk and the hips, deepening the pose.

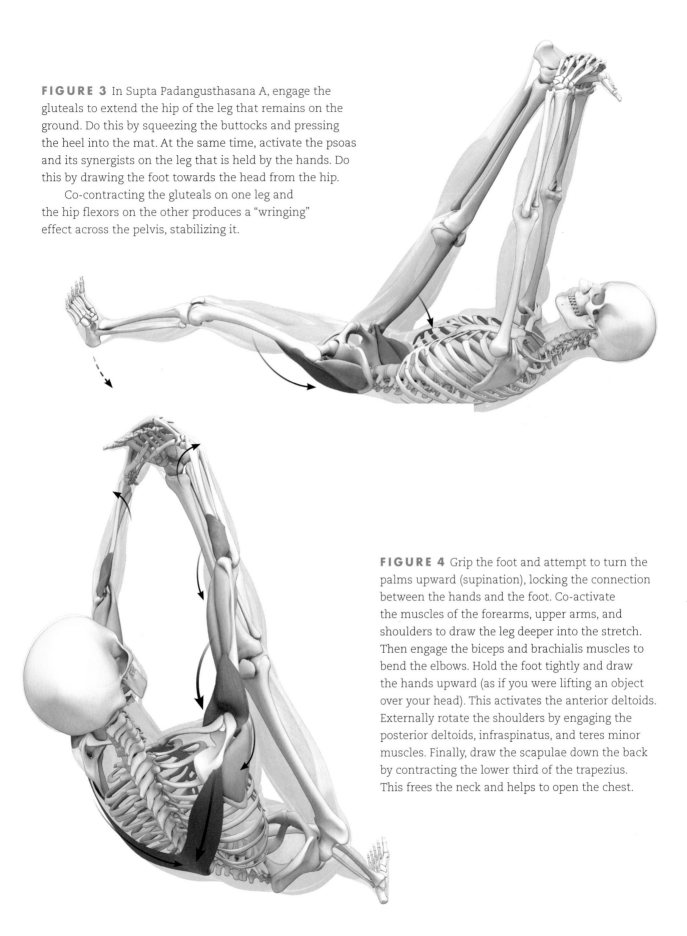

FIGURE 3 In Supta Padangusthasana A, engage the gluteals to extend the hip of the leg that remains on the ground. Do this by squeezing the buttocks and pressing the heel into the mat. At the same time, activate the psoas and its synergists on the leg that is held by the hands. Do this by drawing the foot towards the head from the hip.

Co-contracting the gluteals on one leg and the hip flexors on the other produces a "wringing" effect across the pelvis, stabilizing it.

FIGURE 4 Grip the foot and attempt to turn the palms upward (supination), locking the connection between the hands and the foot. Co-activate the muscles of the forearms, upper arms, and shoulders to draw the leg deeper into the stretch. Then engage the biceps and brachialis muscles to bend the elbows. Hold the foot tightly and draw the hands upward (as if you were lifting an object over your head). This activates the anterior deltoids. Externally rotate the shoulders by engaging the posterior deltoids, infraspinatus, and teres minor muscles. Finally, draw the scapulae down the back by contracting the lower third of the trapezius. This frees the neck and helps to open the chest.

KEY CONCEPT
FACILITATED STRETCHES

FIGURE 1 You can take co-activation a step further by contracting the same muscle that you are attempting to stretch. This eccentric contraction can be used to create length in a muscle, with a technique called facilitated stretching. This utilizes a spinal cord reflex arc and is an example of combining modern Western science with the ancient art of Hatha Yoga. The two go together beautifully. Stretching applies tension to the muscle and its tendon. A nerve receptor (the Golgi tendon organ) is located at the muscle-tendon junction. This receptor senses tension and relays a signal to the spinal cord. The spinal cord then signals the stretching muscle to relax. This reflex arc acts as a protective circuit breaker to prevent the tendon from tearing at its attachment to the bone.

Because all skeletal muscles have Golgi tendon organs, this powerful technique can be applied to gain length and dissolve blockages throughout the body in yoga poses. Use it with caution and care.

FIGURE 1 Spinal Cord Reflex Arc

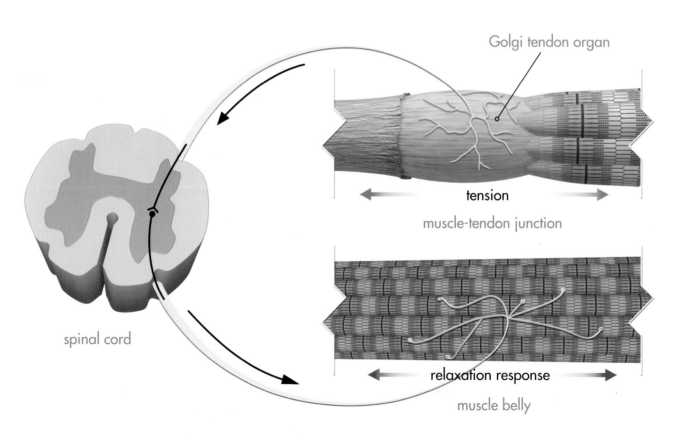

Golgi tendon organ

tension

muscle-tendon junction

relaxation response

muscle belly

spinal cord

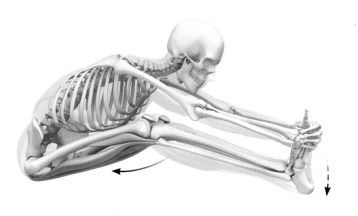

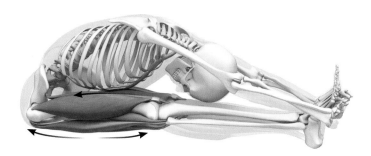

FIGURES 2 & 3 Facilitated stretching involves contracting a muscle that you are lengthening. This increases the tension at the muscle-tendon junction and recruits more Golgi tendon organs than does stretching a muscle alone. Facilitated stretching causes the spinal cord to signal the muscle to relax, in essence, creating "slack" in the muscle. You can then take up the slack to move deeper into the pose.

For example, in Paschimottanasana, slightly bend the knees and squeeze the trunk against the thighs. Then gently press the heels into the mat as if you are trying to flex the knees further. This engages the hamstrings and stimulates the Golgi tendon organs at the muscle-tendon junction. Hold this steady contraction for five to eight breaths before releasing it. This produces relaxation and increased length in the hamstrings. Then contract the quadriceps to straighten the knees and take up the slack created by the reflex arc. This has the added effect of producing reciprocal inhibition, which further relaxes the hamstrings into the stretch.

FIGURES 4 & 5 Follow the same steps in this pose with the quadratus lumborum and erector spinae. First, bend forward to stretch these back muscles. Hold the stretch by bending the arms, and then attempt to arch the back. This increases tension at the muscle-tendon junction of the erector spinae and quadratus lumborum, stimulates the Golgi tendon organs, and ultimately relaxes these muscles. Hold the arch of the back for five to eight smooth breaths. Then engage the abdominals and use the arms to draw yourself deeper into the pose, taking advantage of the new length created by the reflex arc. Activating the abdominals also produces reciprocal inhibition of the back muscles, relaxing them into the stretch.

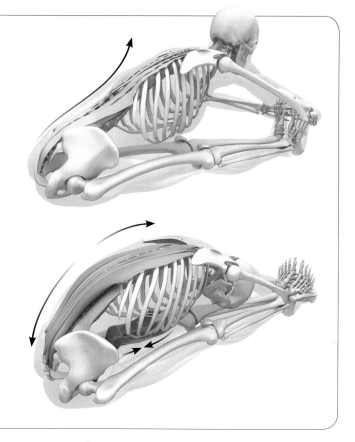

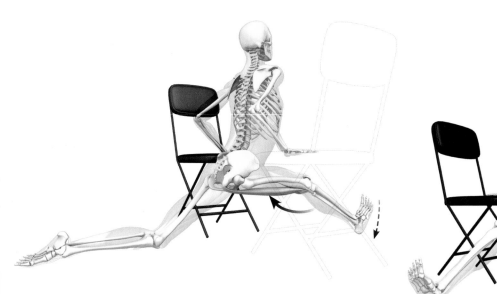

FIGURES 6 & 7 Implement this technique to deepen your Hanumanasana. In the beginning, use a chair on each side of the body for support. Then focus on stretching the forward-leg hamstrings. To do this, flex the forward knee about fifteen degrees. Bending the knee allows you to generate sufficient tension in the stretching hamstrings and protects the joint from hyperextending.

Press the forward-leg heel into the mat to contract the hamstrings. Imagine dragging the heel towards the back knee. Hold this at about twenty percent of your force for several smooth, deep breaths. Then contract the quadriceps to straighten the knee and the psoas to flex the hip. This deepens the pose and takes up the additional length in the muscle produced by the relaxation response.

Next, focus on the back-leg hip flexors. Go into a lunge position to extend the back hip. Then attempt to drag the back knee towards the front foot on the mat (as if you were trying to flex the hip). This augments the tension at the muscle-tendon junction. The mat prevents the knee from moving, but the contraction produced by the effort will stimulate the Golgi tendon organs of the hip flexors. Hold this action for five to eight breaths and release; then take up the slack in these muscles by engaging the back-leg gluteus maximus and hamstrings to extend the hip and deepen the pose.

FIGURE 8 Remember to engage the agonist muscles that produce the form of the pose. In Hanumanasana, contract the forward-leg quadriceps and psoas and the back-leg gluteus maximus and hamstrings. This produces reciprocal inhibition of the muscles we lengthened in the facilitated stretch, allowing them to relax more deeply into the pose.

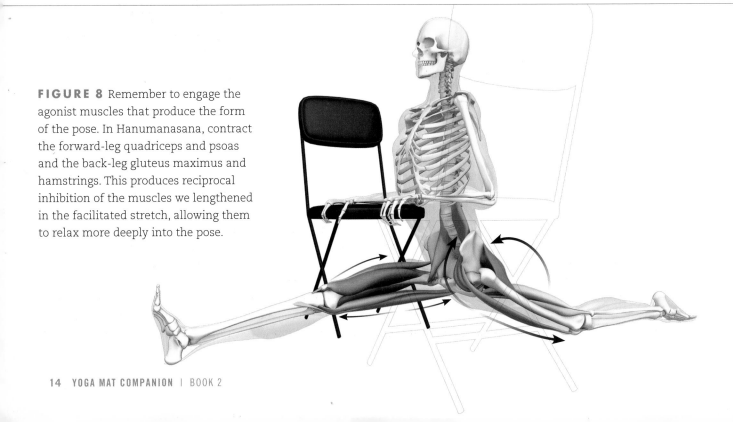

Bandhas stimulate the motor and sensory nerves, creating an imprint of the pose on the brain. They are particularly useful for practitioners who are naturally flexible and can easily attain the form of a pose, yet feel that it is lifeless and has little effect. In such situations, creating a bandha stabilizes the pose and strengthens the muscles. This honors the ha/tha or sun/moon aspect of yoga by balancing flexibility with strength.

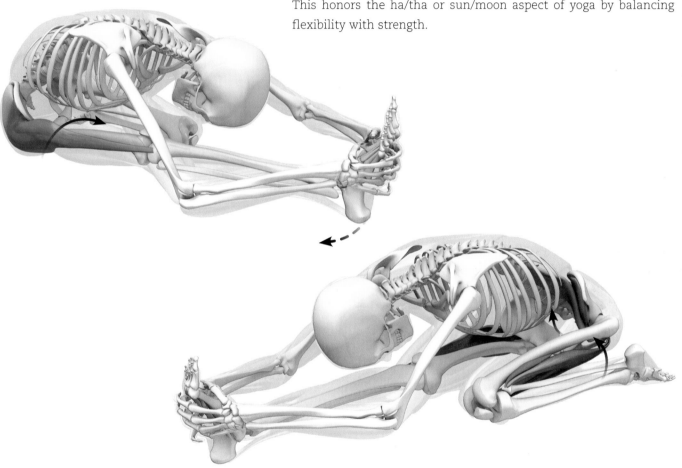

FIGURES 1 & 2 We can use co-contraction to create bandhas. For example, in Triang Mukhaikapada Paschimottanasana there is a tendency to lean or fall over onto the side of the straight leg. One remedy for this is to place a blanket or block under the straight-leg buttocks to shift the weight toward the bent-leg side. Although this can work, it is best to find a way to do the pose without using external props. In this case, we can use muscular forces to counter the tendency to lean over—and at the same time create a bandha in the pose.

Do this by co-contracting the abductor muscles on the straight leg and the hip and knee flexors on the bent leg.

The cue for engaging the abductors is to press the heel into the mat and attempt to drag it outward from the midline. The heel won't move, but the contractile force of the tensor fascia lata and gluteus medius will push the body toward the bent-knee side. At the same time, activate the hamstring muscles to squeeze the calf against the thigh. Then engage the psoas by attempting to lift the bent knee. These actions combine to counteract the tendency to lean toward the straight-leg side. This creates a bandha across the pelvis. Combine these actions with mula bandha by lifting the perineum to engage the muscles of the pelvic floor.

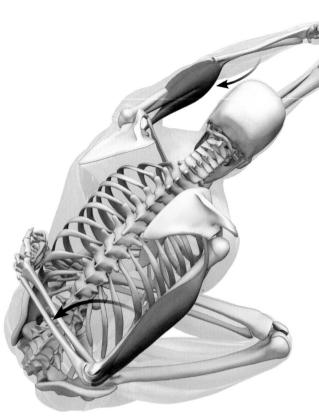

FIGURE 3 Try the following in Ardha Badha Padma Paschimottanasana. Contract the biceps and brachialis muscles to bend the elbow on the side that is grasping the straight-leg foot. Simultaneously attempt to straighten the elbow that is holding the bent-leg foot by engaging the triceps, as shown. Feel the stabilizing effect of co-contracting these muscles. Then add the muscles of the pelvic floor to create mula bandha. Note how activating the biceps and triceps makes it easier to engage the muscles of the pelvic floor—a process known as recruitment.

FIGURE 4 There are several bandhas available in Padmasana, or Lotus Pose. Try these and feel how the pose comes alive, especially if Lotus is easy for you. Begin by pressing the lower-side leg against the upper side (where the lower legs cross). This engages the gluteus maximus and deep external rotators of the lower-side hip. At the same time, press the top leg into the lower one. This activates the gluteus medius and tensor fascia lata of the top leg. Feel how this stabilizes the pose.

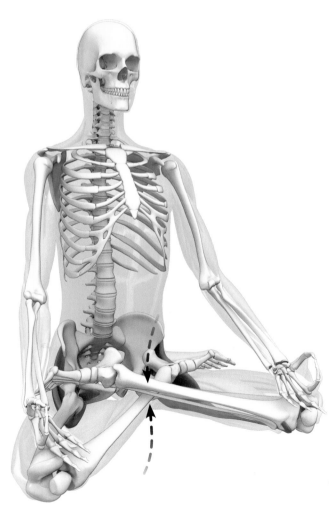

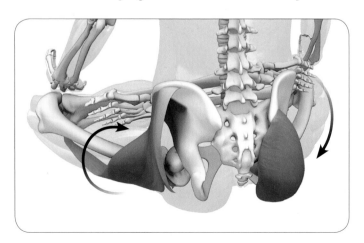

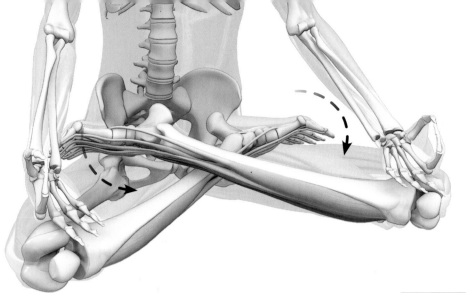

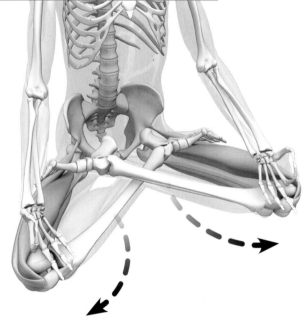

◀ FIGURE 5 Next, hook the tops of the feet over the thighs by contracting the peroneus longus and brevis muscles on the sides of the lower legs, as well as the tibialis anterior and toe extensors. This holds the feet in place.

▶ FIGURE 6 With the feet constrained on the thighs (as illustrated in Figure 5), attempt to straighten the knees by engaging the quadriceps. The quadriceps are muscular stabilizers of the knees. Contracting them in Lotus solidifies the pose and maintains congruency of the knee joint. This helps to protect against injury to the cartilage.

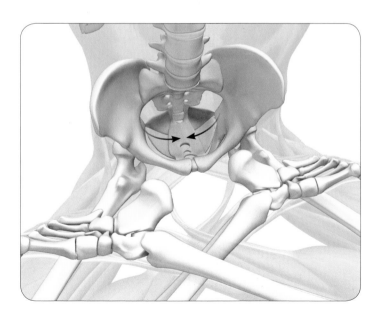

FIGURE 7 Finally, engage the muscles of the pelvic floor to activate mula bandha. A cue for this is to perform the Kegel maneuver. Note how combining the bandhas described above with mula bandha strengthens it. This is due to recruitment. Engaging easy-to-access muscles adds to the force of muscles that are harder to contract at will (such as those that create mula bandha).

SUMMARY We can see from this section that the concept of a *lock* or *bandha* can be extended beyond the more familiar mula, udyana, and jalandhara bandhas. In fact, you can use co-activation of muscle groups to create bandhas throughout the body in yoga poses. These locks can be employed to stabilize articulations, stimulate spinal cord reflex arcs, and enable movement in relatively immobile regions, such as the sacroiliac joint.

THE BANDHA YOGA CODEX

EACH YOGA POSTURE HAS ITS OWN UNIQUE FORM AND FUNCTION. MUSCLES THAT engage in one posture may be stretching in another. For this reason it helps to have a road map for navigating your way to the optimal pose. Better still is the ability to create your own road map. The Bandha Yoga Codex shows you how to do this.

There are five elements to every asana. These are the joint positions, the muscles that engage to produce these positions, the muscles that stretch, the breath, and the bandhas. Understanding the joint positions enables you to determine the muscles that produce the posture. Engage the prime movers to sculpt the pose, and polish it with the synergists. Once you know the prime movers, you can identify the muscles that are stretching. Apply physiological techniques to lengthen these muscles and create mobility to deepen the pose.

Then there is the breath. In virtually every posture we can benefit from expanding the chest. Combine the accessory muscles of breathing with the action of the diaphragm to increase the volume of the thorax. This improves oxygenation of the blood and removes energetic blockages in the subtle body.

The bandhas are the finishing touch. Co-activate the muscle groups that produce the joint positions and you will create bandhas throughout the body. Then connect these peripheral locks to the core bandhas. This produces stability in the pose and accentuates the sensory imprint of the asana on the mind.

The Bandha Yoga Codex is a five-step process that teaches how to identify these elements and decode any pose. This is your guide to creating a road map for combining science and yoga. I use Janu Sirsasana to illustrate the Codex on the following pages.

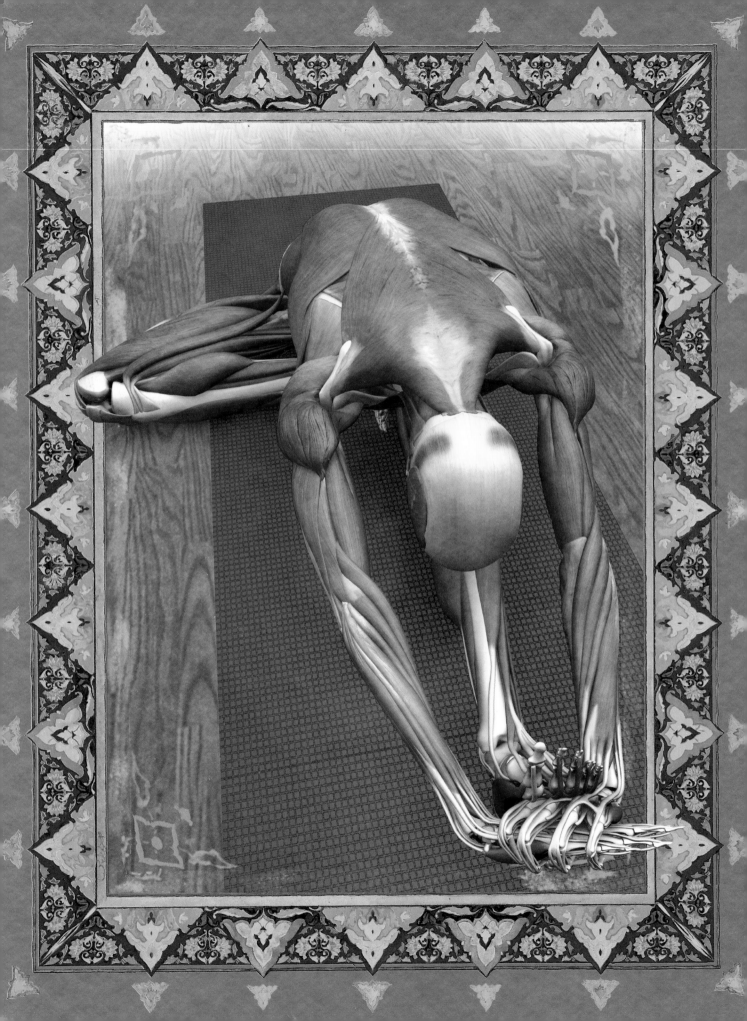

बन्ध योग

The Bandha Yoga Codex

— 1 —

Define the position of the joints in the pose.

— 2 —

Identify the prime mover muscles that act
on the joints to create the pose.
Contract these muscles to align and
stabilize the skeleton.

— 3 —

Identify the antagonist muscles
of the prime movers.
Stretch these muscles to create flexibility.

— 4 —

Expand the chest.

— 5 —

Create a Bandha.

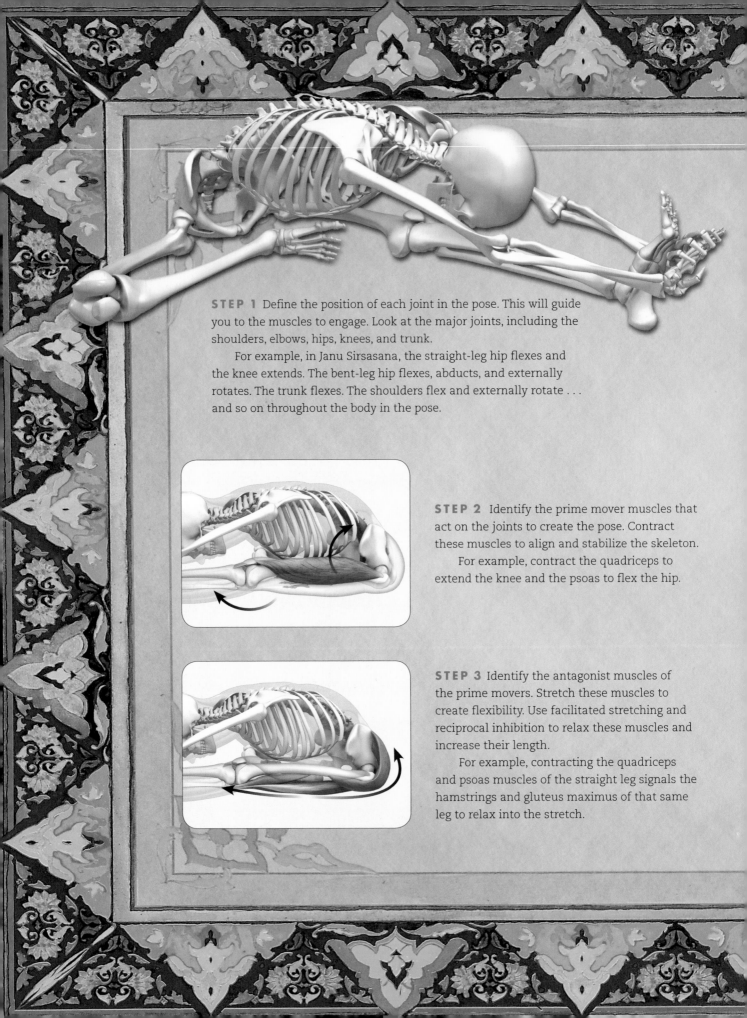

STEP 1 Define the position of each joint in the pose. This will guide you to the muscles to engage. Look at the major joints, including the shoulders, elbows, hips, knees, and trunk.

For example, in Janu Sirsasana, the straight-leg hip flexes and the knee extends. The bent-leg hip flexes, abducts, and externally rotates. The trunk flexes. The shoulders flex and externally rotate . . . and so on throughout the body in the pose.

STEP 2 Identify the prime mover muscles that act on the joints to create the pose. Contract these muscles to align and stabilize the skeleton.

For example, contract the quadriceps to extend the knee and the psoas to flex the hip.

STEP 3 Identify the antagonist muscles of the prime movers. Stretch these muscles to create flexibility. Use facilitated stretching and reciprocal inhibition to relax these muscles and increase their length.

For example, contracting the quadriceps and psoas muscles of the straight leg signals the hamstrings and gluteus maximus of that same leg to relax into the stretch.

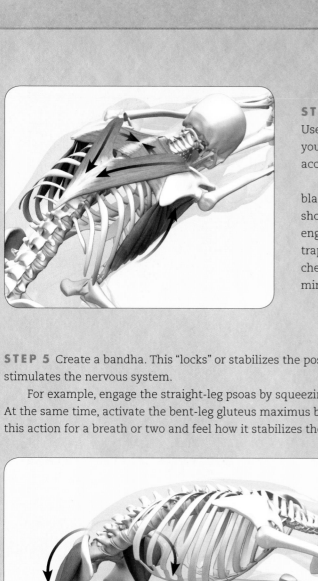

STEP 4 Expand the chest. Use the cues in this book to train yourself to isolate and engage the accessory muscles of breathing.

For example, draw the shoulder blades toward the midline and the shoulders away from the ears by engaging the rhomboids and lower trapezius. Then lift and expand the chest by contracting the pectoralis minor and serratus anterior muscles.

STEP 5 Create a bandha. This "locks" or stabilizes the pose, strengthens the muscles, and stimulates the nervous system.

For example, engage the straight-leg psoas by squeezing the torso against the thigh. At the same time, activate the bent-leg gluteus maximus by contracting the buttocks. Hold this action for a breath or two and feel how it stabilizes the pelvis in Janu Sirsasana.

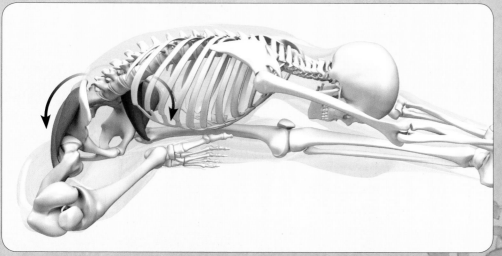

HIP OPENERS

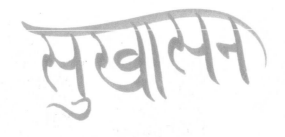

SUKHASANA

EASY CROSS-LEGGED POSE

SUKHASANA IS THE SEATED POSITION MOST COMMONLY USED IN MEDITATION. Accordingly, many of the other poses of Hatha Yoga are directed toward making it easier and more comfortable to sit for long periods in this pose. In fact, the Sanskrit word *asana* is often translated to mean "a comfortable and easy position."

To sit comfortably in Sukhasana, we want to minimize the muscular effort required to be in the pose. One way to achieve this is by bringing the knees closer to the mat, thereby lowering the center of gravity toward the pelvic core. Do this by stretching the muscles that surround the hips, especially the adductors and internal rotators. This allows the femurs to abduct and externally rotate.

Align the vertebral column over the pelvis so that the weight of the trunk is supported by the skeleton (bones) instead of primarily by muscular contraction. This makes it possible to hold the pose with less effort. Use closed chain contraction of the latissimus dorsi to draw the torso forward so that the mechanical axis (the direction of gravity) and the anatomical axis of the vertebral column align with each other. Refine the pose by engaging the accessory muscles of breathing to expand the chest.

BASIC JOINT POSITIONS

- The hips flex, abduct, and externally rotate.
- The knees flex.

- The ankles are neutral.
- The trunk extends slightly.
- The shoulders flex slightly.

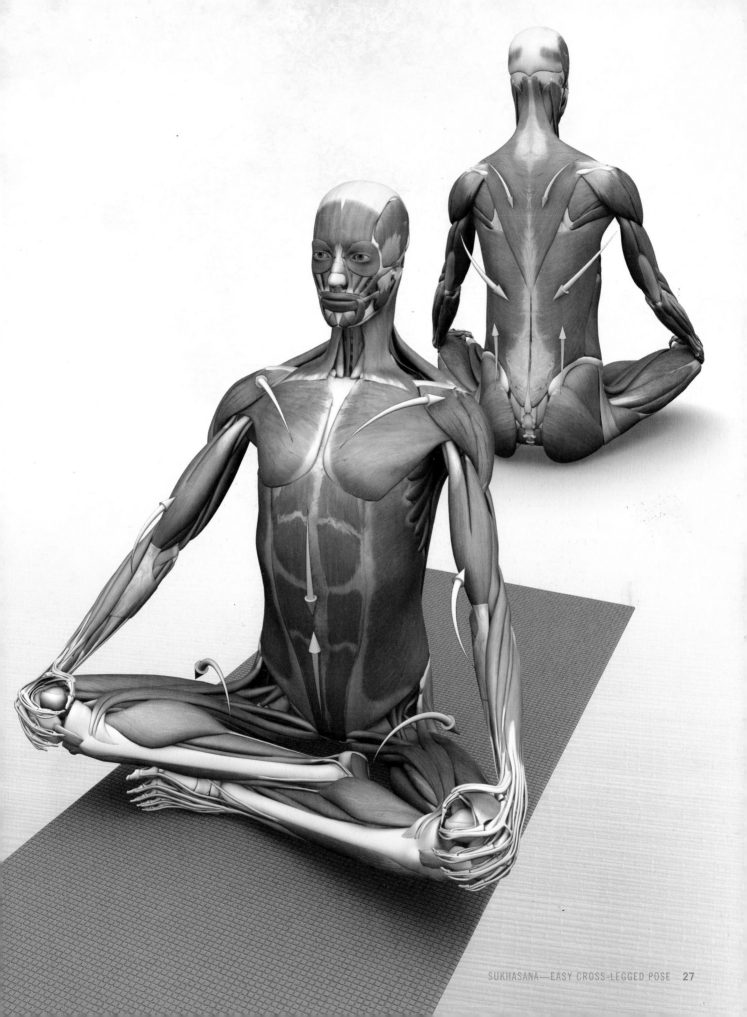

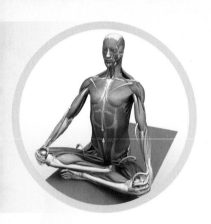

Sukhasana Preparation

Stretch the adductor group on the insides of the thighs with poses such as Baddha Konasana and Upavistha Konasana. Use facilitated stretching to lengthen the internal rotators with the cradle stretch.

Lift the chest by fixing the hands on the knees and attempting to pull back. The arms will not move so the chest is drawn forward by closed chain contraction of the latissimus dorsi. This draws the vertebral column over the pelvis and expands the chest.

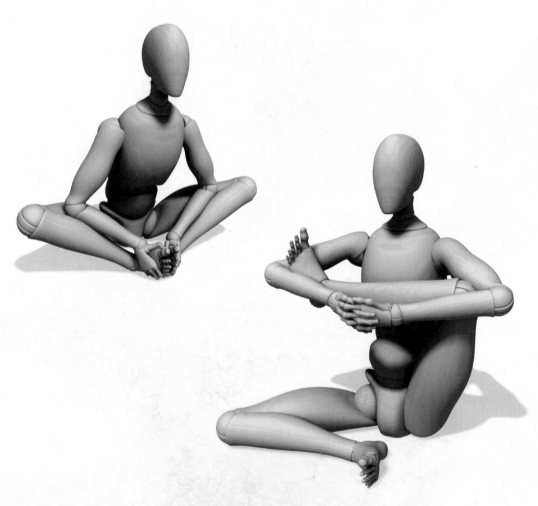

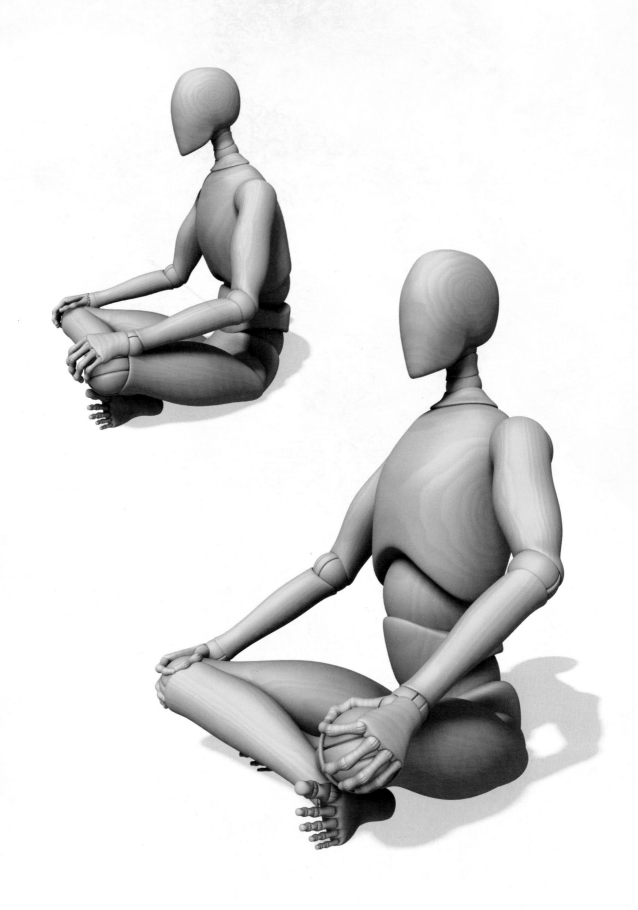

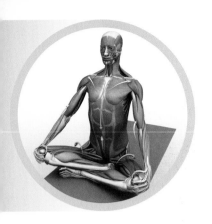

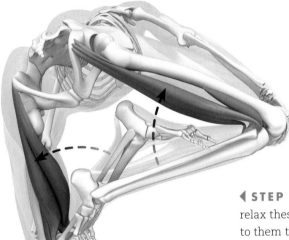

▶ STEP 1 Activate the psoas muscles by pressing down on the knees while trying to lift them. This produces a closed chain contraction, whereby the origin of the psoas moves (not the insertion), lifting the lumbar and tilting the pelvis forward. This synergizes the action of the quadratus lumborum on the lumbar spine. Visualize the sartorius contracting to flex, abduct, and externally rotate the hips. This muscle also assists the psoas in tilting the pelvis forward.

◀ STEP 2 Bend the knees by engaging the hamstrings. We relax these muscles once in the pose but occasionally return to them to refine the position of the legs and re-establish congruency of the knee joints.

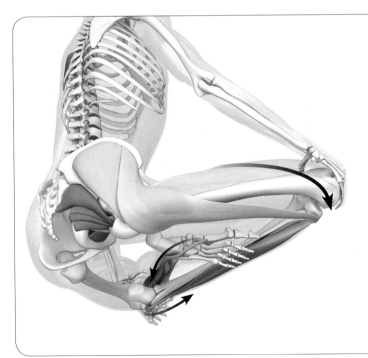

STEP 3 The tensor fascia lata and gluteus medius activate to abduct the thighs toward the floor. Note that these muscles are internal rotators of the hips. Sukhasana *externally* rotates the hips. Accordingly, prepare for the pose by stretching the tensor fascia lata and gluteus medius to lengthen their internal rotation components. Then engage the same muscles to abduct the hips.

Tuck the tailbone while turning the thighs outward to engage the deep external hip rotators. Refine the pose by gently pressing the outer edges of the feet into the mat. This activates the peroneus longus and brevis muscles at the sides of the lower legs.

▶ **STEP 4** Place the hands on the knees and pronate the forearms to turn the palms down, engaging the pronators teres and quadratus. Contract the triceps to attempt to straighten the elbows. Engage the infraspinatus and teres minor muscles to externally rotate the shoulders. The posterior deltoids synergize this action. Then pull with the hands to draw the chest forward, activating the latissimus dorsi in a closed chain fashion, as shown.

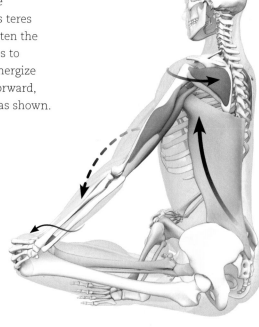

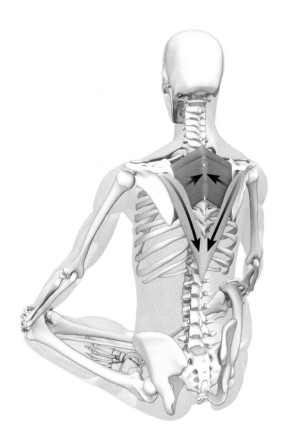

◀ **STEP 5** Draw the shoulder blades toward the midline by contracting the rhomboids. This opens the chest and stabilizes the scapulae in place, preparing for Step 6. Activate the lower third of the trapezius to draw the shoulder blades down the back.

▶ **STEP 6** Stabilize the scapulae toward the midline of the back. Then lift the ribcage by engaging the pectoralis minor. The cue for activating this muscle is to attempt to roll the shoulders forward. Because the shoulders are fixed in place by the rhomboids, they will not actually roll forward. Instead, the contraction of the pectoralis minor lifts the ribs and opens the chest.

Expand the chest further by engaging the serratus anterior. Note how this muscle also originates from the scapula and attaches to the ribs (like the pectoralis minor). Accordingly, when the scapulae are tethered in place by the rhomboids, engaging the serratus anterior lifts and expands the chest. The cue for contracting this muscle is to visualize pressing the hands outward against a door frame.

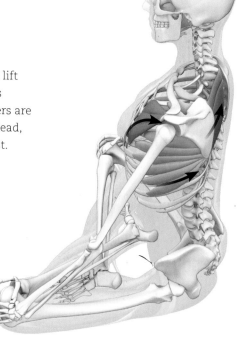

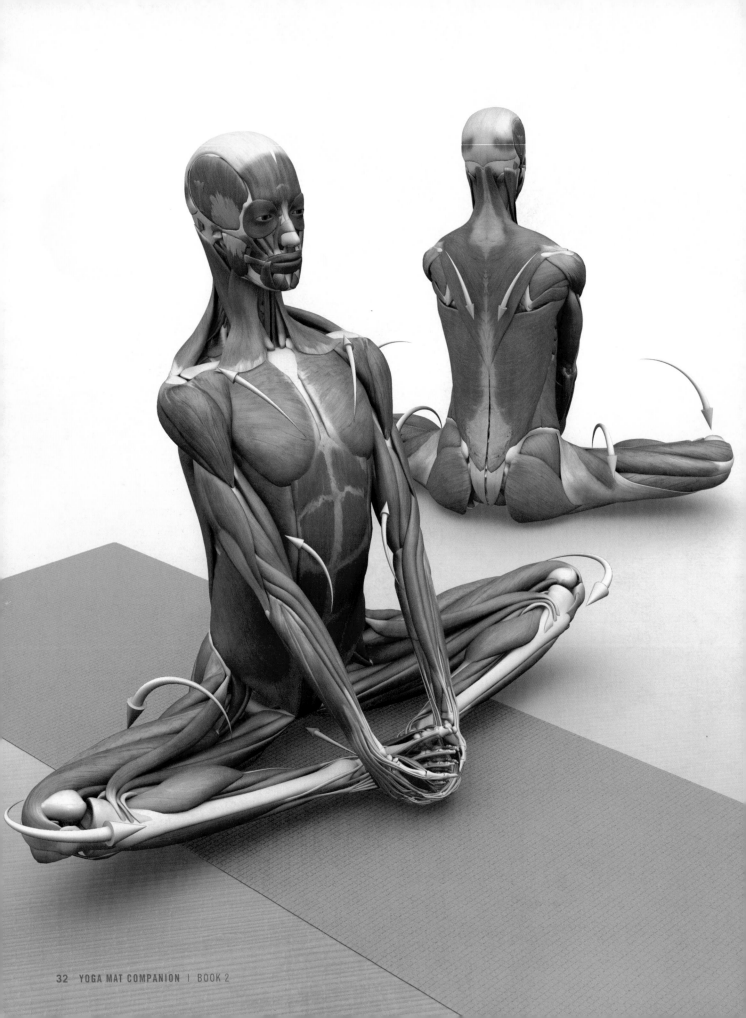

बद्धकोणासन

BADDHA KONASANA
BOUND ANGLE POSE

BADDHA KONASANA IS A SYMMETRICAL POSE. AS SUCH, IT PROVIDES AN OPPORTUNITY for locating and balancing asymmetries, particularly in the hips and pelvis. First identify the elemental movements that create the form of the pose. For example, the hips flex, abduct, and externally rotate. Each component of hip movement is like a subplot in the story of the pose. Focusing on specific components brings greater awareness to the nuances of each movement. Begin with abduction: tight adductors can restrict drawing the knees apart. Use facilitated stretching, as detailed in the Key Concepts, to create length in the adductor group and free the hips to open the knees. Then work on improving external rotation of the hips. Limitations in this movement may stem from tightness in the internal rotators—the gluteus medius and minimus and the tensor fascia lata. Use the facilitated stretch provided for Padmasana (Lotus Pose) to increase the range of hip external rotation. Combine this with the mobility gained in abduction to deepen Baddha Konasana.

Next, invoke the deep external rotators of the hip and the muscles of the pelvic floor to nutate the sacrum and gain subtle depth in the pose. Connect the hands and feet. One variation has the elbows bending to draw the body forward. In another variation, the back arches and the shoulder blades draw together to lift the torso upward, expanding the chest. Use the arms in combination with the hamstrings to draw the feet closer to the pelvis—one objective of the final pose. Remember to maintain the knees as hinge joints. Gain most of your mobility from the hips, which are ball and socket joints.

BASIC JOINT POSITIONS

- The hips flex, abduct, and externally rotate.
- The knees flex.
- The ankles are neutral.

- The trunk extends.
- The shoulders flex, adduct, and externally rotate.
- The elbows flex.

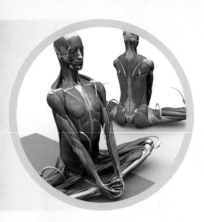

Baddha Konasana Preparation

Bend the knees and take the general shape of the pose by flexing, abducting, and externally rotating the hips. Squeeze the lower legs against the thighs to activate the hamstrings. The hamstrings are muscular stabilizers of the knees; engaging them maintains congruency of the knee joint and helps to prevent excessive force being transmitted to the articular cartilage of the knee. Grasp the feet with the hands, and place the elbows into the crease between the upper and lower legs. Attempt to close (adduct) the knees to engage the adductor muscles in a facilitated stretch. Use a maximum of twenty percent of your force to draw the legs against the arms. Hold this action for a few slow, deep, and steady breaths. Then release the contraction and draw the knees closer to the floor by engaging the muscles at the sides of the hips—the gluteus medius and tensor fascia lata. This takes up the slack produced by the facilitated stretch and creates a new set length for the adductor muscles. Lengthen the internal rotators of the hips using the cradle stretch to increase external rotation. Repeat again as necessary to increase mobility of the hips. Carefully release the pose. Take Dandasana to contract and balance the muscles you have just stretched in Baddha Konasana— the adductors and internal rotators of the hips. This maintains the ha/tha or yin/yang nature of yoga.

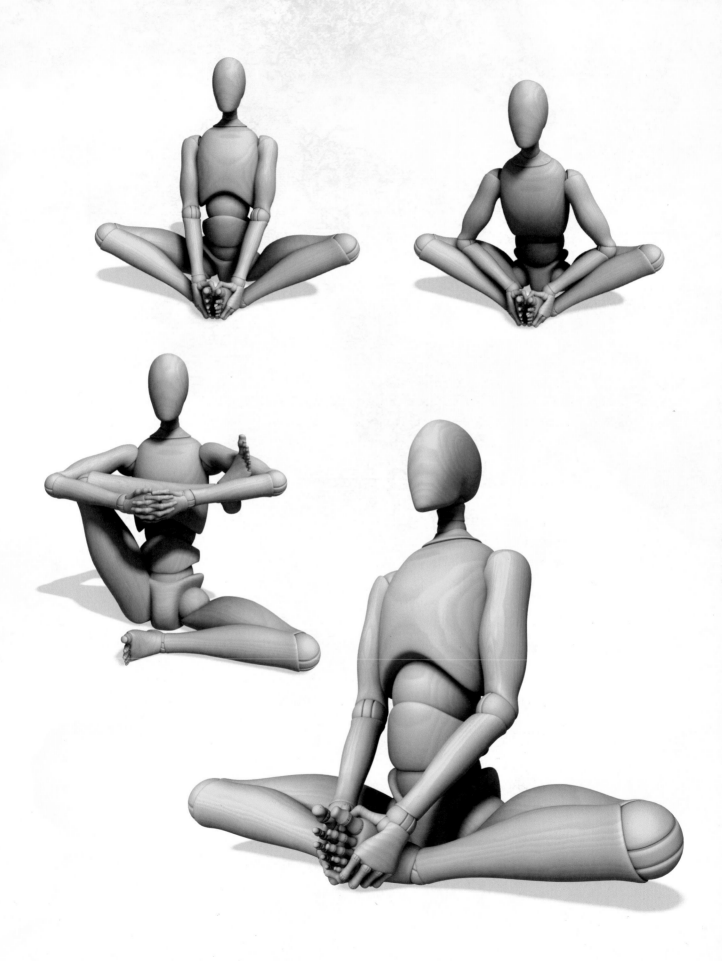

BADDHA KONASANA—BOUND ANGLE POSE **35**

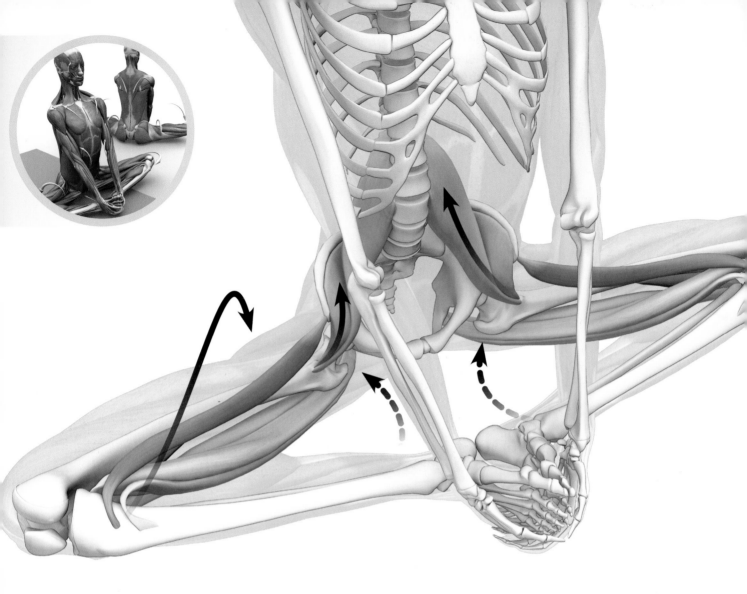

STEP 1 Flex the knees by engaging the hamstrings. Contracting the hamstrings not only bends the knees but also tucks the tailbone under, because the hamstrings originate from the ischial tuberosities on the back of the pelvis. Remember that the hips externally rotate in Baddha Konasana; tucking the tailbone under turns the hips outward and synergizes external rotation. The sartorius muscle runs from the front of the pelvis to the inner knee. It flexes, abducts, and externally rotates the hip. When contracted, the sartorius feels like a cord at the front of the pelvis. Its name derives from the Latin for "tailor," because tailors used to sit cross-legged while they worked. Note that this muscle also crosses the knee and thus aids the hamstrings in flexing and stabilizing this joint in the pose.

Engage the psoas to flex and externally rotate the hips. A cue for this action is to press the hands on the knees and then attempt to draw them toward the body while resisting with the hands.

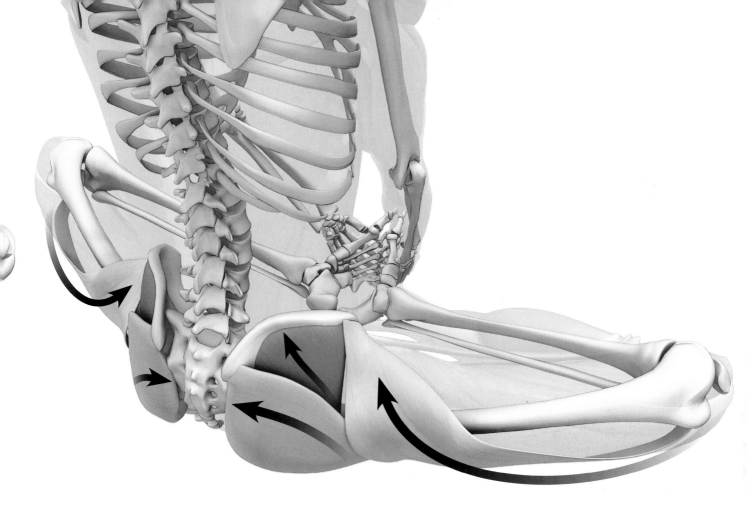

STEP 2 Squeeze the sides of the buttocks to abduct and externally rotate the hips, drawing the knees toward the floor. The gluteus maximus externally rotates the hips while the gluteus medius and tensor fascia lata abduct them. Activating these muscles stimulates reciprocal inhibition of the adductor group on the inner thighs, allowing them to relax into the stretch. You may note the paradox in contracting the gluteus medius and tensor fascia lata, since they also internally rotate the hips. In Baddha Konasana, the primary action of these muscles is to abduct the femurs. Certain fibers of these muscles must also be stretched to allow for the external rotation, as described in the preparation.

Note that when the hips are fully abducted, the contractile force of the tensor fascia lata and gluteus medius is far less, because these muscles are shortened almost completely. At this point it becomes necessary to engage the hamstrings and use the hands to draw the feet closer to the pelvis and the knees closer to the floor. The gluteus medius, tensor fascia lata, and gluteus maximus (the fibers that attach to the iliotibial band) act together to provide that extra inch of abduction in the pose. (The iliotibial band is a fibrous ribbon-like tendon that runs from the upper thigh to just below the knee. Both the tensor fascia lata and the gluteus maximus insert onto it. It abducts the hip and stabilizes the knee.)

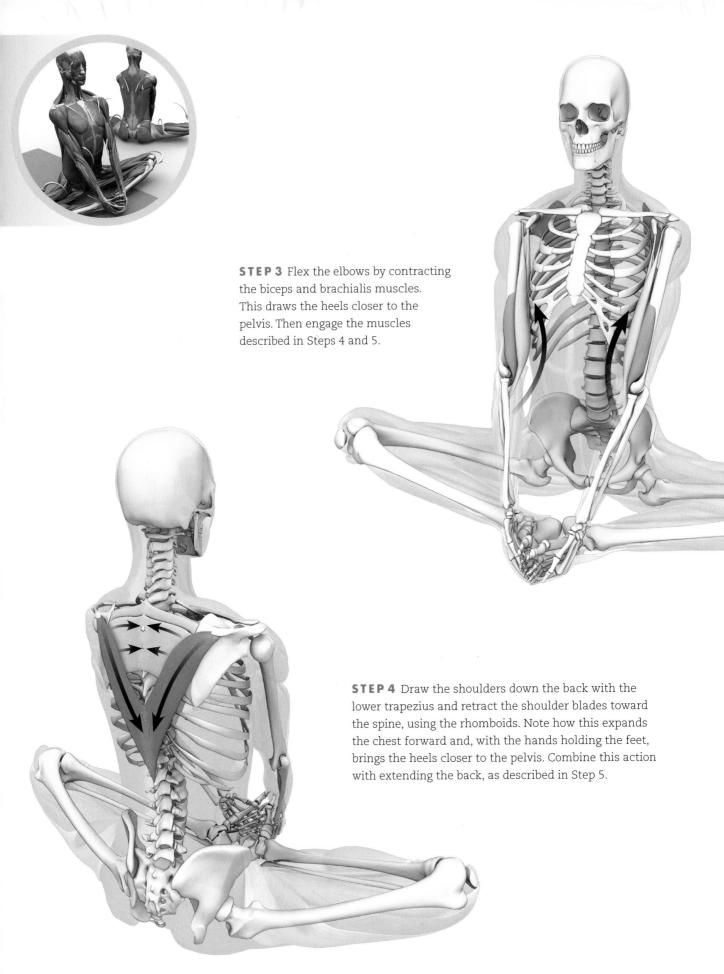

STEP 3 Flex the elbows by contracting the biceps and brachialis muscles. This draws the heels closer to the pelvis. Then engage the muscles described in Steps 4 and 5.

STEP 4 Draw the shoulders down the back with the lower trapezius and retract the shoulder blades toward the spine, using the rhomboids. Note how this expands the chest forward and, with the hands holding the feet, brings the heels closer to the pelvis. Combine this action with extending the back, as described in Step 5.

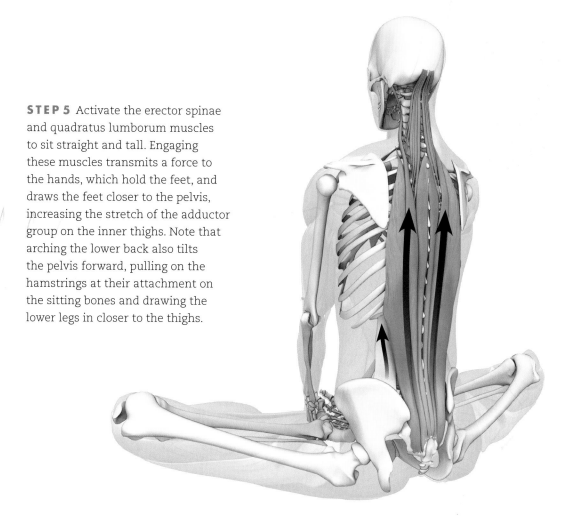

STEP 5 Activate the erector spinae and quadratus lumborum muscles to sit straight and tall. Engaging these muscles transmits a force to the hands, which hold the feet, and draws the feet closer to the pelvis, increasing the stretch of the adductor group on the inner thighs. Note that arching the lower back also tilts the pelvis forward, pulling on the hamstrings at their attachment on the sitting bones and drawing the lower legs in closer to the thighs.

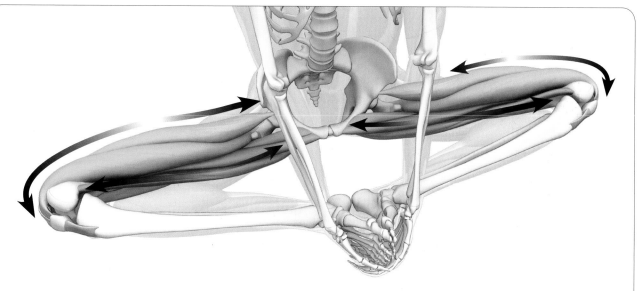

SUMMARY All of these interrelating subplots of the pose combine to stretch the adductor muscles on the inner thighs and the fibers of the gluteus medius, gluteus minimus, and tensor fascia lata that internally rotate the hips. Remember to balance this stretch by returning to Dandasana after the pose, and feel how practicing Baddha Konasana improves your Dandasana.

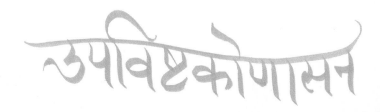

UPAVISTHA KONASANA

WIDE-ANGLE SEATED FORWARD BEND POSE

COMPARE UPAVISTHA KONASANA WITH BADDHA KONASANA AND PASCHIMOTTANASANA. Look at the similarities and differences that make each pose unique in form and function. For example, Baddha Konasana flexes, abducts, and externally rotates the hips. Although Upavistha Konasana is similar in this respect, the knees extend and the trunk flexes forward as in Paschimottanasana. Note that when the hips are fully flexing, as in Upavistha Konasana, the prime movers of this action are in a state of active insufficiency; that is, the contractile elements of the psoas and its synergists cannot generate significant increased force to deepen the pose. You can, however, take advantage of the psoas muscle being polyarticular (crossing multiple joints); it runs from the lumbar spine and across the sacroiliac joint and front of the pelvis to insert onto the femur. Engage the abdominals to slightly round the back; this lengthens the psoas major out to a point where contracting it will generate force to further flex the hips. Use the hands and arms to fix the hips in this new, more deeply flexed position, and then activate the erector spinae and quadratus lumborum muscles to arch the lower back.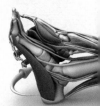

To review, when a muscle is fully contracted, it cannot generate much force to deepen the pose. However, polyarticular muscles such as the psoas can move multiple joints along their length. This means that they can be stretched at one point and then contracted further along at another. Additionally, Upavistha Konasana connects the hands and feet to maintain and increase hip and trunk flexion.

BASIC JOINT POSITIONS

- The hips flex, abduct, and externally rotate.
- The knees extend.
- The ankles are neutral.
- The feet evert.
- The trunk flexes forward.

- The cervical spine extends.
- The shoulders extend, abduct, and externally rotate.
- The elbows flex.
- The wrists flex.

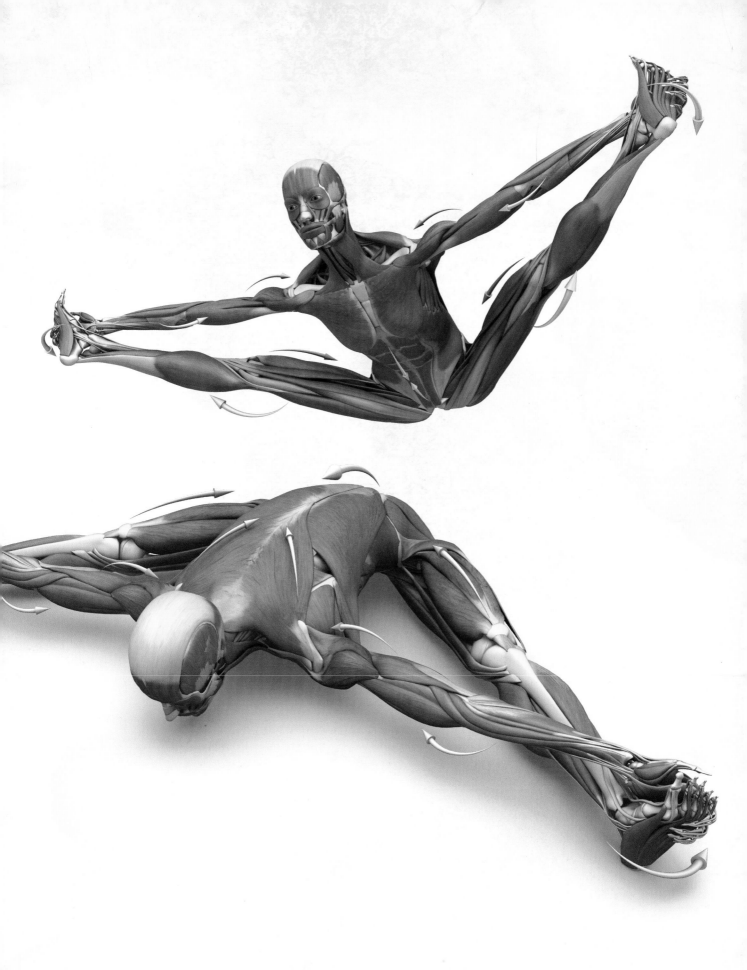

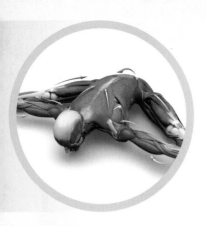

Upavistha Konasana Preparation

Begin by linking the upper and lower extremities. If you cannot reach the feet with the hands, use belts. Bend the knees to release the hamstrings at their insertions on the lower legs. Draw the trunk down towards the floor. This moves the origins of the hamstrings at the ischial tuberosities up and back, taking up the slack in these muscles created by bending the knees. Then straighten the knees to take the hamstrings out to length at their insertions, and feel the stretch. Bend the elbows to pull yourself forward.

As you gain flexibility, toss the belts aside and reach forward to take the feet, bending the knees once again to release the hamstrings. Hold on tight with the hands, and then straighten the knees to pull the trunk forward.

Plan your exit from Upavistha Konasana by bending the knees. Then consciously engage the lower back muscles to sit up. Use the hands to adduct the legs back to the midline, and take Dandasana. This balances the intense hip abduction and trunk flexion of Upavistha Konasana with adduction and mild spinal extension, respectively. Stabilize your body first and come out of the pose with grace and control.

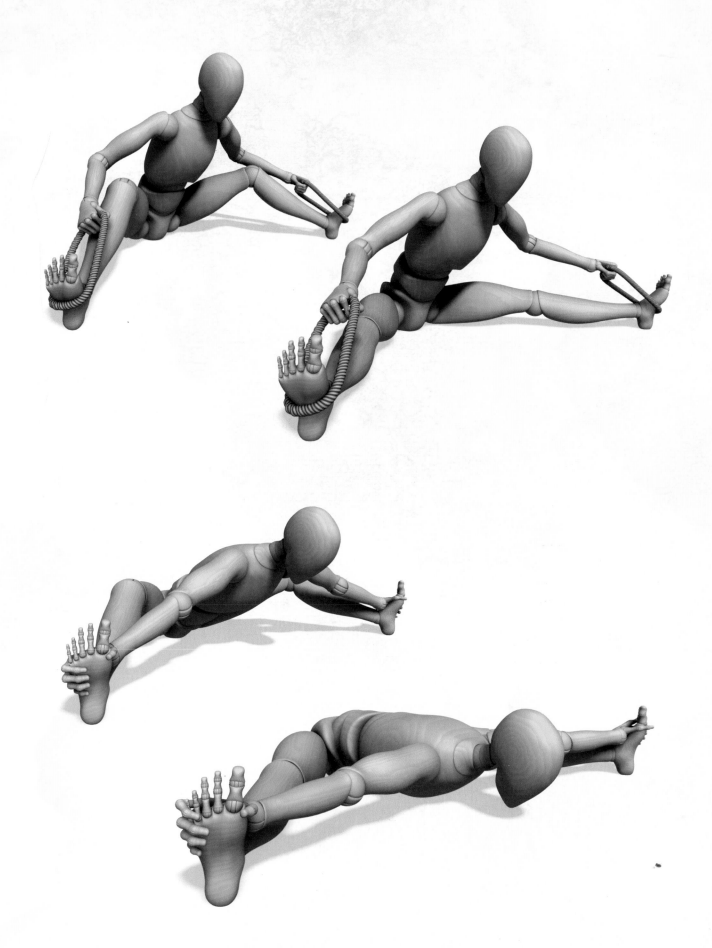

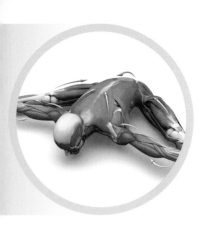

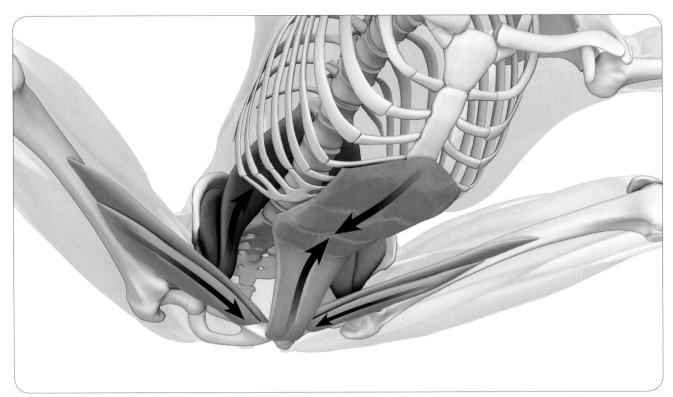

▲ **STEP 1** Once you are in the general form of the pose, use your knowledge of biomechanics to deepen it in precise and meticulous ways. Surprising energetic openings can take place in millimeters gained on the physical level. For example, when the psoas is in a fully contracted state, it cannot generate additional force to flex the trunk further. It must first be taken out to length to regain contractile ability. Gain this length by engaging the rectus abdominis to flex the lumbar spine. Then contract the psoas to draw the trunk deeper into the pose.

The adductors longus and brevis and the pectineus are synergists of the psoas for hip flexion. A cue for activating these muscles is to fix the feet on the mat and attempt to "scrub" them toward one another. The mat prevents the feet from moving, but the action engages the hip flexors. Feel how you move deeper into the pose with this cue.

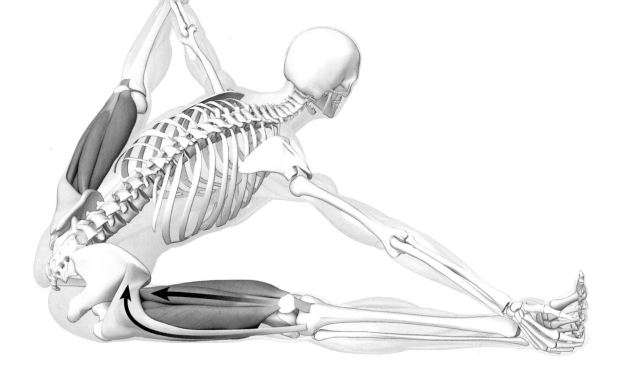

▲ **STEP 2** Straighten the knees and draw the kneecaps up by contracting the quadriceps. This takes the hamstrings out to length from their insertions on the lower legs and also stimulates reciprocal inhibition of these muscles, allowing them to relax. Consciously relax them as well. Engage the gluteus medius and tensor fascia lata to draw the legs away from the midline (abduction). Note that when you stretch a muscle, it will pull on the bone at its insertion. This is why stretching the gluteus maximus often results in external rotation of the thigh. Counter this by turning the thighs inward so that the kneecaps face up. Remember that the hip abductors, the tensor fascia lata and gluteus medius, also internally rotate the thighs. Engage them to create this action. The tensor fascia lata synergizes the quadriceps in straightening the knees.

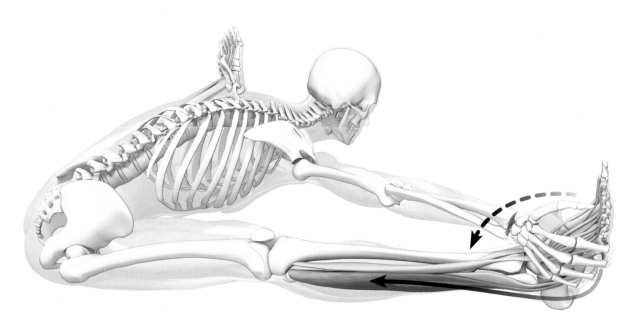

▲ **STEP 3** Evert the soles of the feet by tilting the feet outward, activating the peroneus longus and brevis muscles. Contract the long and short toe extensors to lift the toes. Dynamize the arches by engaging the tibialis posterior muscles, and feel how these actions combine to stabilize the ankles and open the soles of the feet.

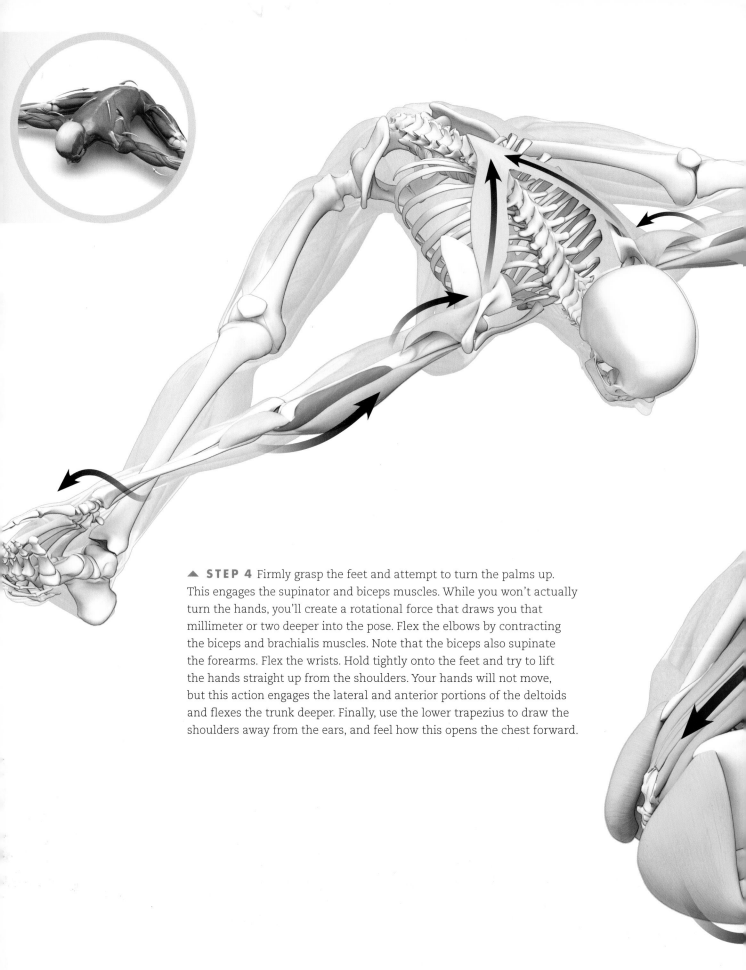

▲ **STEP 4** Firmly grasp the feet and attempt to turn the palms up. This engages the supinator and biceps muscles. While you won't actually turn the hands, you'll create a rotational force that draws you that millimeter or two deeper into the pose. Flex the elbows by contracting the biceps and brachialis muscles. Note that the biceps also supinate the forearms. Flex the wrists. Hold tightly onto the feet and try to lift the hands straight up from the shoulders. Your hands will not move, but this action engages the lateral and anterior portions of the deltoids and flexes the trunk deeper. Finally, use the lower trapezius to draw the shoulders away from the ears, and feel how this opens the chest forward.

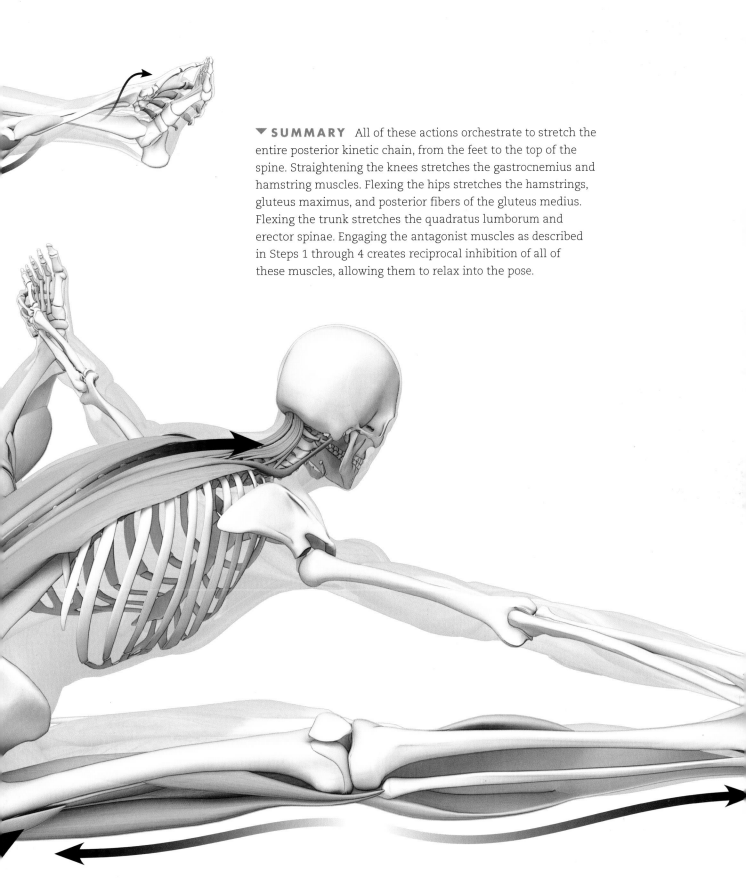

▼ **SUMMARY** All of these actions orchestrate to stretch the entire posterior kinetic chain, from the feet to the top of the spine. Straightening the knees stretches the gastrocnemius and hamstring muscles. Flexing the hips stretches the hamstrings, gluteus maximus, and posterior fibers of the gluteus medius. Flexing the trunk stretches the quadratus lumborum and erector spinae. Engaging the antagonist muscles as described in Steps 1 through 4 creates reciprocal inhibition of all of these muscles, allowing them to relax into the pose.

SUPTA PADANGUSTHASANA B

SLEEPING BIG-TOE POSE VERSION B

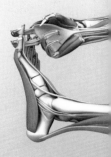

SUPTA PADANGUSTHASANA B FLEXES, ABDUCTS, AND EXTERNALLY ROTATES THE hip of the lifted leg and straightens the knee. If we straighten the knee more or flex the leg up higher, we intensify the stretch of the hamstrings. This is an example of triangulation, wherein the origin of the hamstrings on the ischial tuberosity represents one point of the triangle and the insertion on the lower leg represents another. The hamstrings are the apex or focal point. Actions that move the origins and insertions farther away from one another conspire to stretch the hamstrings. Externally rotating the thigh preferentially lengthens the semimembranosus and semitendinosus (the inside hamstrings).

The shoulder and arm perform a secondary action that affects the focal point of this story. If you lift the arm and attempt to bend the elbow, you can draw the leg up higher. The trunk assists in this action when we slightly arch the back and rotate away from the lifted leg.

Then there is the leg that remains extended along the mat. The foot of this leg tends to lift off the floor and externally rotate. Use coupled joint movements to address this: extend the lumbar spine and hip to bring the foot back to the ground. Then press the heel into the mat and attempt to drag it to the side. This cue engages the muscles that turn the thigh inward, countering the external rotation of the leg.

BASIC JOINT POSITIONS

- The hip of the leg on the mat extends and internally rotates.
- The hip of the held leg flexes, abducts, and externally rotates.
- The knees extend.
- The trunk extends and the cervical spine rotates.

- The shoulder on the held-leg side abducts and externally rotates.
- The elbow extends.
- The other shoulder adducts and internally rotates.
- The elbow flexes slightly.
- The forearm pronates.

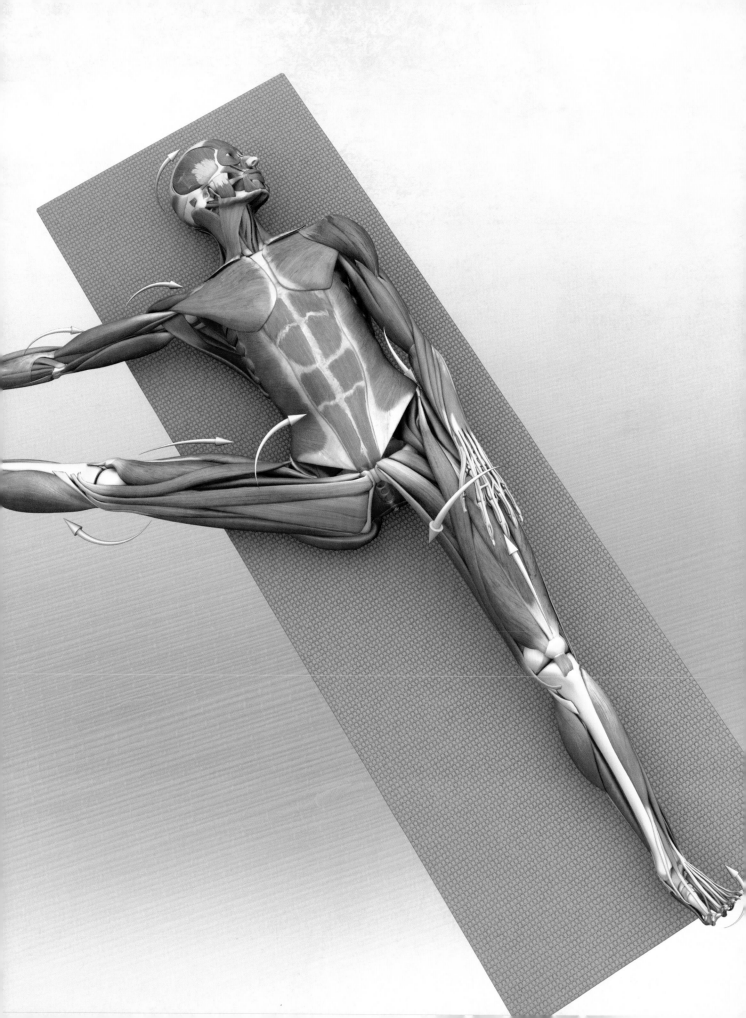

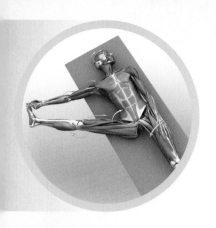

Supta Padangusthasana B
Preparation

If you're unable to reach the foot, use a belt to tether the abducted leg. With increased flexibility, grasp the big toe with the thumb and first two fingers.

Feel how bending the elbow or lifting the arm increases the stretch at the back of the leg. Keep the other leg bent in the beginning, and rest the palm on the thigh. Then straighten the knee and extend the hip by contracting the quadriceps, gluteals, and lower back muscles. Press the hand into the front of the thigh to further stabilize the leg.

Add Trikonasana in the preparation to stretch the hamstrings from a different orientation and to improve your understanding of the interrelatedness of the poses.

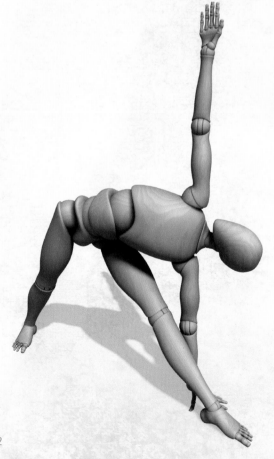

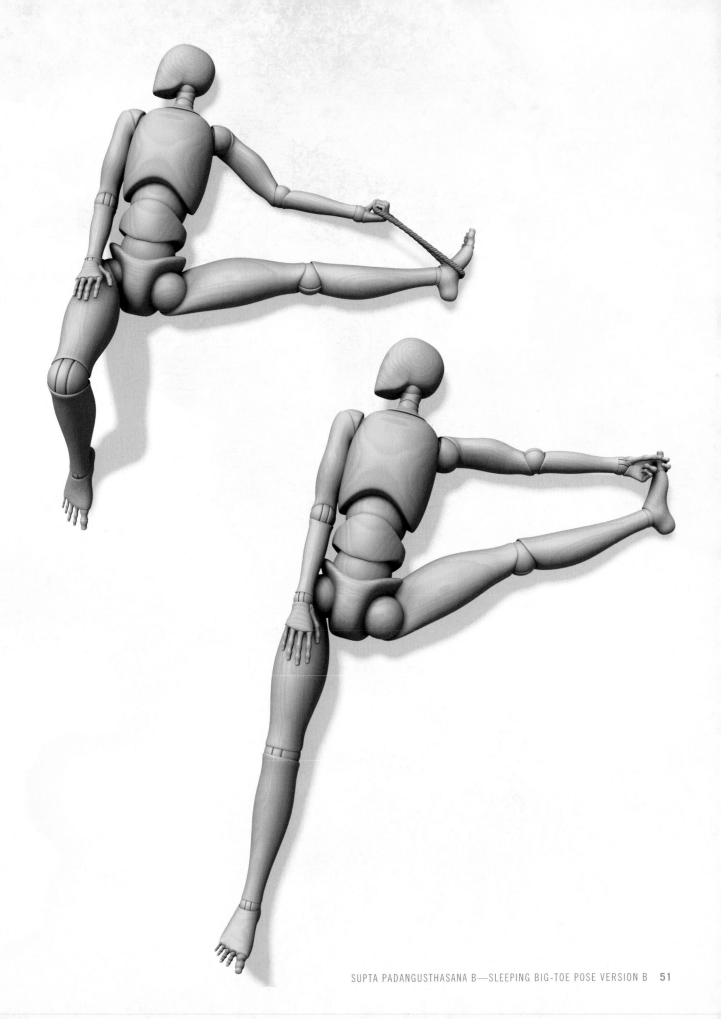

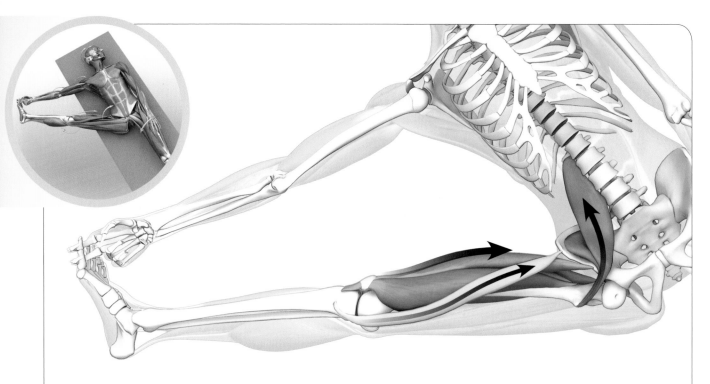

STEP 1 Flex and externally rotate the hip of the lifted leg, using the psoas and its synergist, the sartorius. Note how the psoas wraps over the front of the pelvis. Contracting this muscle tilts the pelvis forward, while at the same time flexing and externally rotating the femur. This is an example of coupled joint movement. Engage the quadriceps to straighten the knee.

STEP 2 Use the muscles that abduct and elevate the shoulder— the upper pectoralis major and the lateral deltoids—to lift the foot. Once you feel these muscles contract, focus on them to refine and stabilize the lift. Externally rotate the forearm by engaging the supinator muscle and slightly bend the elbow by contracting the biceps and brachialis. These actions in the upper extremity combine to lift the leg, illustrating how to use muscles that are distant from the targeted joint (here, the hip) to move that joint.

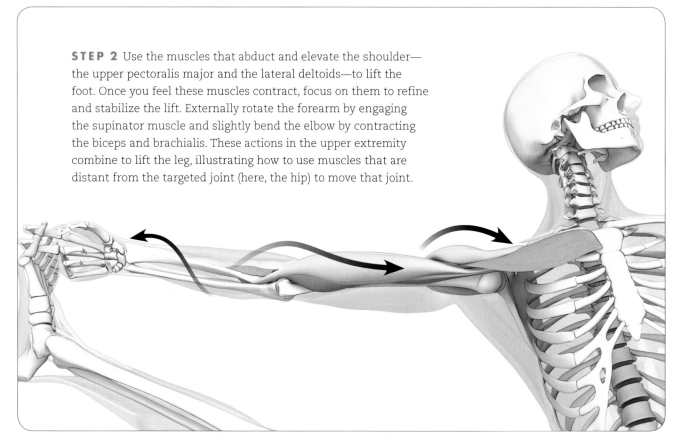

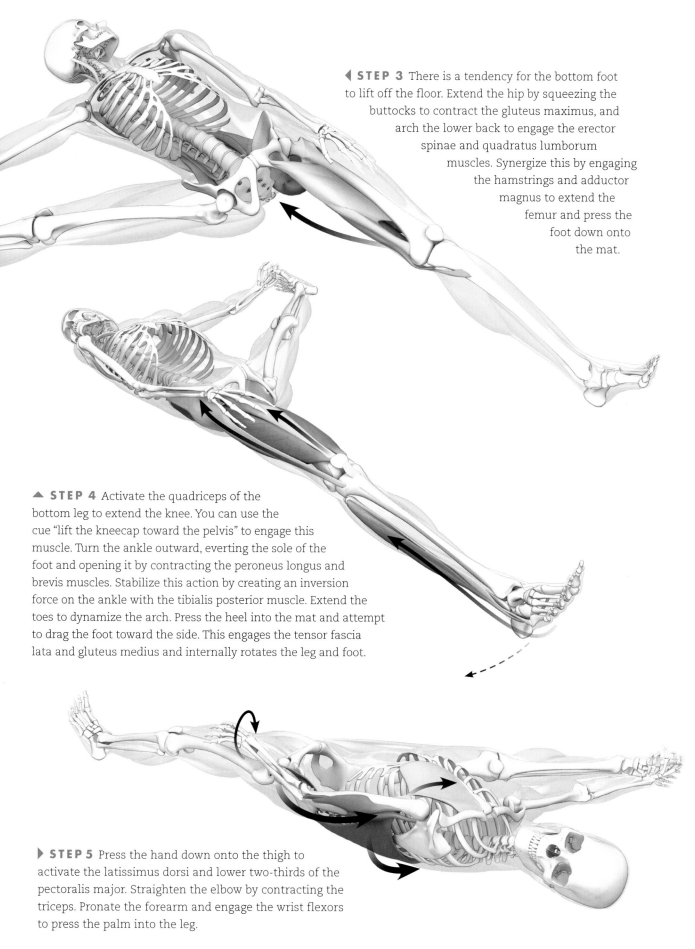

STEP 3 There is a tendency for the bottom foot to lift off the floor. Extend the hip by squeezing the buttocks to contract the gluteus maximus, and arch the lower back to engage the erector spinae and quadratus lumborum muscles. Synergize this by engaging the hamstrings and adductor magnus to extend the femur and press the foot down onto the mat.

STEP 4 Activate the quadriceps of the bottom leg to extend the knee. You can use the cue "lift the kneecap toward the pelvis" to engage this muscle. Turn the ankle outward, everting the sole of the foot and opening it by contracting the peroneus longus and brevis muscles. Stabilize this action by creating an inversion force on the ankle with the tibialis posterior muscle. Extend the toes to dynamize the arch. Press the heel into the mat and attempt to drag the foot toward the side. This engages the tensor fascia lata and gluteus medius and internally rotates the leg and foot.

STEP 5 Press the hand down onto the thigh to activate the latissimus dorsi and lower two-thirds of the pectoralis major. Straighten the elbow by contracting the triceps. Pronate the forearm and engage the wrist flexors to press the palm into the leg.

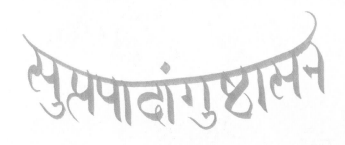

SUPTA PADANGUSTHASANA

SLEEPING BIG-TOE POSE, BENT-KNEE VERSION

IN THIS VERSION OF SUPTA PADANGUSTHASANA, WE COMPLETELY FLEX THE hip of the leg that is held in the hands. This focuses the stretch on the gluteus maximus and proximal hamstrings—the portion of the muscle group that is closer to the origin on the sitting bones. Grasp the foot and flex the elbows to draw the foot deeper into the armpit and increase the stretch in the buttocks; this is the main story of the pose. Contracting the abdominals flexes the trunk, creating a secondary action that deepens the main stretch. Engage the gluteals of the straight leg to extend the hip and the quadriceps to straighten the knee. The foot will tend to externally rotate due to the action of the gluteus maximus. Oppose this tendency by turning the thigh inward. This is easier said than done, so in the muscles section, we offer a technique to accomplish this.

BASIC JOINT POSITIONS

- The hip of the leg on the floor extends and internally rotates.
- The knee extends.
- The foot everts.
- The toes extend.
- The hip of the held leg flexes and adducts.
- The knee flexes.
- The trunk flexes.
- The shoulders flex, abduct, and externally rotate.
- The elbows flex.
- The forearms supinate.
- The wrists flex.

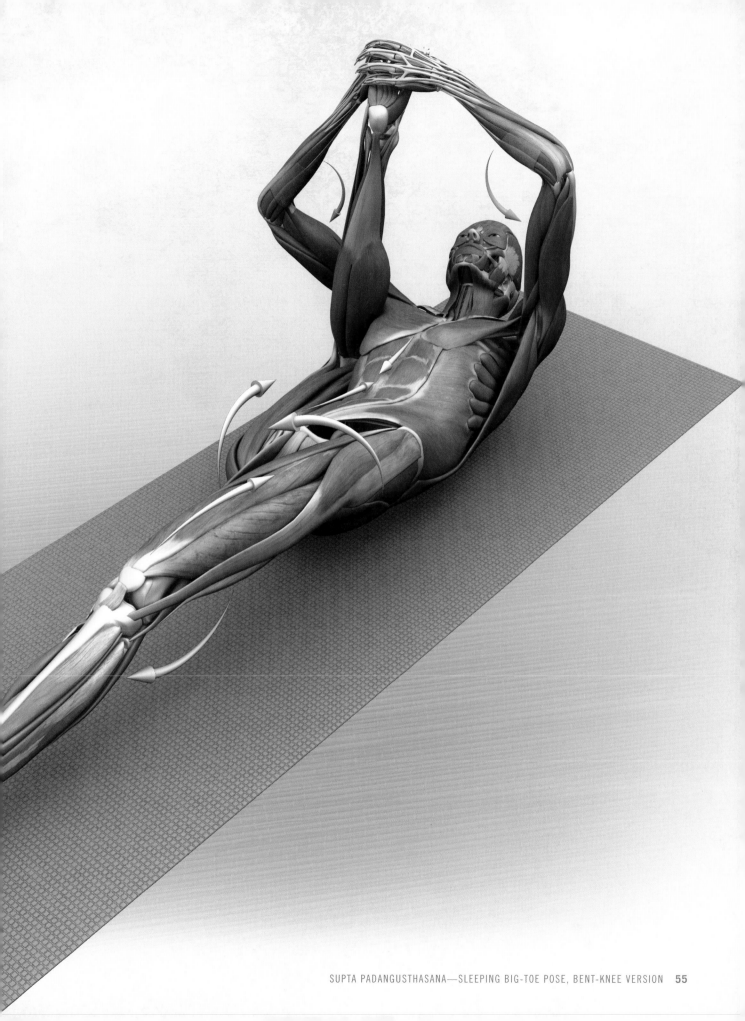

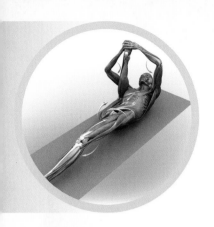

Supta Padangusthasana Preparation

In the beginning, use a belt to tether the upper-leg foot and maintain the bottom leg bent, as shown. There are stretch receptors in the muscle belly called muscle spindles that detect changes in length and tension. When a muscle stretches, these receptors initiate a signal from the central nervous system that tells the muscle to contract to protect itself. Engaging the muscles that produce the general form of the pose causes the muscle spindle to acclimate. The contractile signal from the spinal cord then decreases, allowing relaxation into the pose. As you become more flexible, grasp the foot with the hands. Bend the elbows so that the force of contracting the biceps is directed down through the long axis of the tibia. Now straighten the bottom leg and extend the hip to complete the asana.

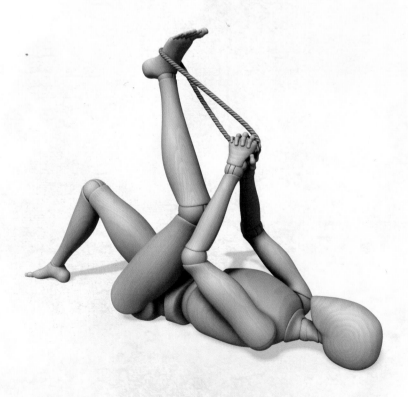

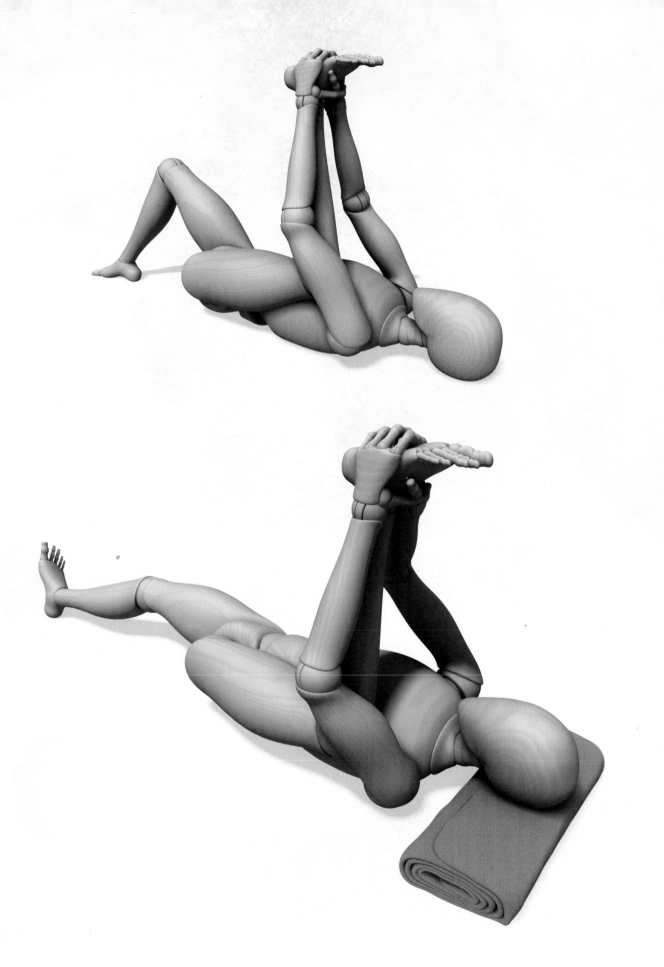

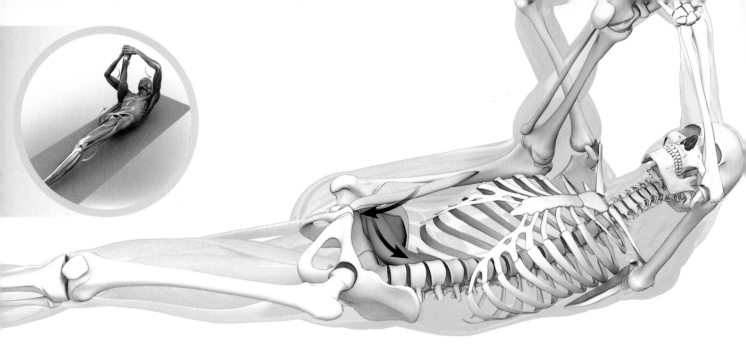

▲ STEP 1 Use the psoas and its synergists, the pectineus and adductors longus and brevis, to initiate flexion of the hip. Note that once you are deep within the pose, these muscles have minimal impact on increasing this action. Because there is maximum overlap of the cross-bridges in the muscles, they are incapable of generating much, if any, additional contractile force. At this point, the hip is further flexed by the action of the upper extremities pulling down through the foot.

▶ STEP 2 Grasp the foot with both hands and imagine raising the arms overhead in front of you. Use this cue to activate the anterior deltoids, which flex the shoulders and thereby draw the hip deeper into the pose. Then bend the elbows by contracting the biceps and brachialis muscles. Align the hands so that the direction of the force from bending the elbows is drawn down through the long axis of the tibia.

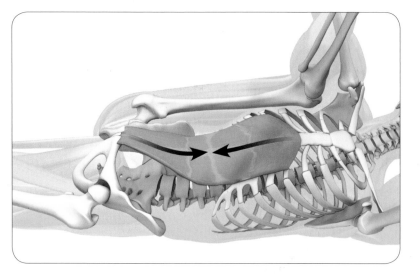

◀ STEP 3 Hold the foot with the hands and contract the rectus abdominis to flex the trunk toward the thigh, pulling the foot deeper into the armpit. Fix the foot in this position with the arms and follow the instructions in Step 4.

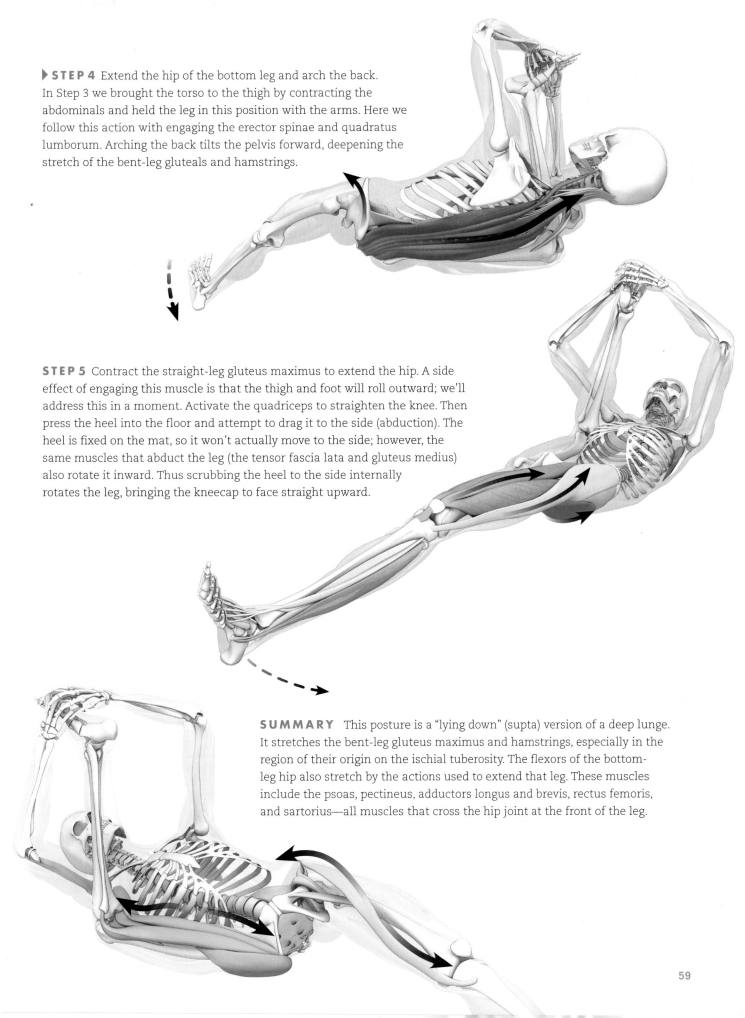

▶ **STEP 4** Extend the hip of the bottom leg and arch the back. In Step 3 we brought the torso to the thigh by contracting the abdominals and held the leg in this position with the arms. Here we follow this action with engaging the erector spinae and quadratus lumborum. Arching the back tilts the pelvis forward, deepening the stretch of the bent-leg gluteals and hamstrings.

STEP 5 Contract the straight-leg gluteus maximus to extend the hip. A side effect of engaging this muscle is that the thigh and foot will roll outward; we'll address this in a moment. Activate the quadriceps to straighten the knee. Then press the heel into the floor and attempt to drag it to the side (abduction). The heel is fixed on the mat, so it won't actually move to the side; however, the same muscles that abduct the leg (the tensor fascia lata and gluteus medius) also rotate it inward. Thus scrubbing the heel to the side internally rotates the leg, bringing the kneecap to face straight upward.

SUMMARY This posture is a "lying down" (supta) version of a deep lunge. It stretches the bent-leg gluteus maximus and hamstrings, especially in the region of their origin on the ischial tuberosity. The flexors of the bottom-leg hip also stretch by the actions used to extend that leg. These muscles include the psoas, pectineus, adductors longus and brevis, rectus femoris, and sartorius—all muscles that cross the hip joint at the front of the leg.

सुतपादांगुष्ठासन श्री

SUPTA PADANGUSTHASANA A

SLEEPING BIG-TOE POSE VERSION A

SUPTA PADANGUSTHASANA A STRETCHES THE HAMSTRINGS, GASTROCNEMIUS, AND gluteus maximus of the leg that is held in the air. Use the weight of the torso to draw the leg deeper into the stretch, while at the same time engaging the quadriceps to straighten the knee and create reciprocal inhibition of the hamstrings.

This is a good pose in which to apply facilitated stretching. Do this by holding the foot firmly by the heel, and then attempt to bend the knee, eccentrically contracting the hamstrings. This stimulates the Golgi tendon organ, a sensory receptor located at the muscle-tendon junction. The Golgi tendon organ then signals the spinal cord that there is increased tension, and the spinal cord completes the feedback loop by signalling the hamstrings to relax into the stretch. This is part of the complex system that controls muscle tension and length. Use this technique carefully (see page 12 for a reference on facilitated stretching). Although the main story of this pose is the stretch at the back of the held leg, a subplot exists in the leg that remains on the mat. Notice the challenge of keeping the hip extended, the thigh inwardly rotated, and the heel on the floor. Yet this is the form of the pose we want to work toward. Use the muscles of the buttocks and lower back to draw the heel down, and use the internal rotators of the hip to bring the kneecap facing straight up. We explain this technique in the muscles section.

BASIC JOINT POSITIONS

- The hip of the leg on the floor extends and internally rotates.
- The held-leg hip flexes.
- The knees extend.
- The held-leg ankle plantar flexes.
- The feet evert and the toes extend.
- The trunk flexes.
- The shoulders flex, adduct, and externally rotate.
- The elbows flex.
- The forearms supinate.
- The wrists flex.

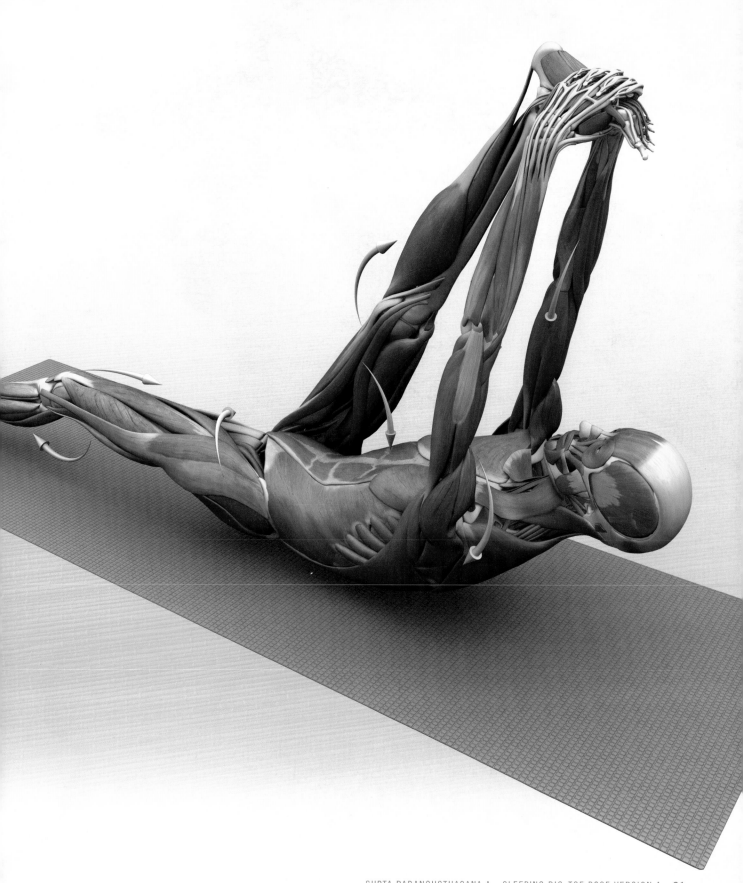

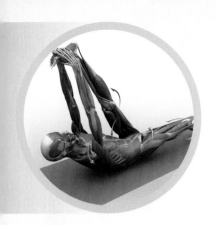

Supta Padangusthasana A
Preparation

Use a belt to grasp the foot as shown. Bend the elbows to draw the leg closer. Do not rush or force the stretch, as this can damage the hamstrings. When you're flexible enough, you can reach up and take the foot or lower leg with the hands. Grasping the foot, use the shoulder muscles to attempt to lift the arms upward toward the head and draw the leg deeper into the stretch. During this time you can keep the other knee bent. For the final pose, straighten the knee and internally rotate the thigh of the leg that remains on the floor.

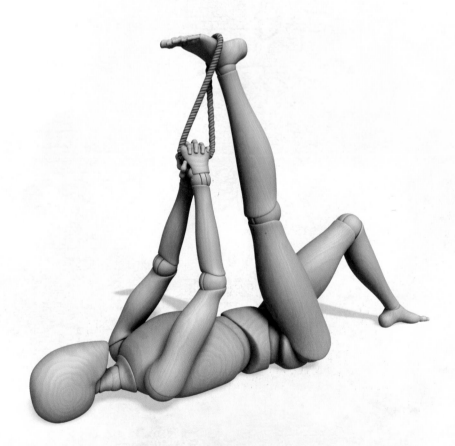

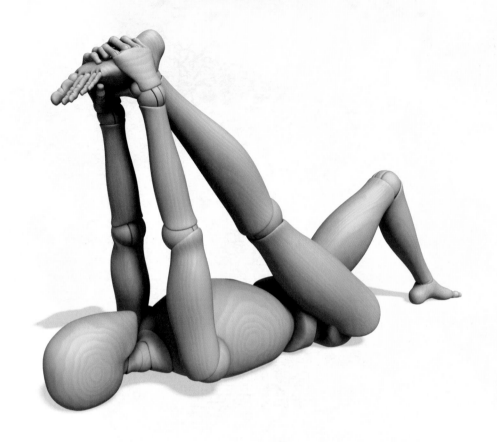

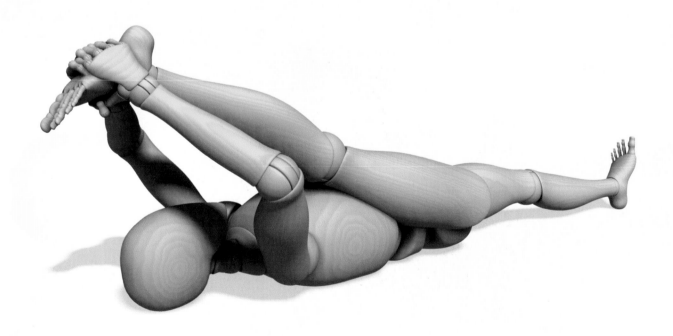

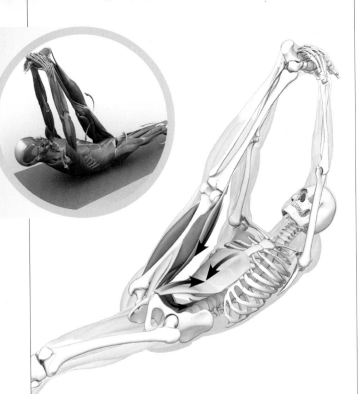

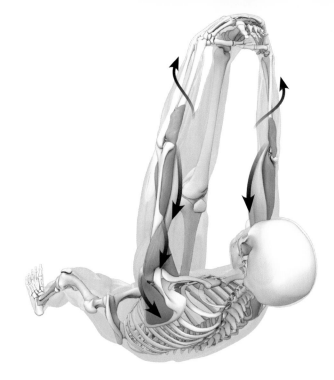

STEP 1 Activate the hip flexors, including the psoas, pectineus, and adductors longus and brevis, to bring the leg up. Notice that when the hip is fully flexed, these muscles can generate very little force because they are beyond their optimal contractile length. Squeeze the abdomen to flex the trunk toward the leg, and contract the quadriceps to straighten the knee. This initiates reciprocal inhibition of the muscles that are lengthening and allows them to relax into the stretch.

▲ **STEP 2** Grasp the foot with the hands and attempt to raise the arms over the head. This engages the anterior deltoids and draws the leg deeper into the stretch. Externally rotate the shoulders by activating the infraspinatus and teres minor muscles of the rotator cuff. Flex the elbows to draw the leg deeper into the stretch by engaging the biceps and brachialis muscles. Supinate the forearms by attempting to turn the palms up while holding the foot. This adds a "helical" force from the feet to the shoulders through the elbows, creating a wringing effect that stabilizes the foot and draws the leg deeper into the pose.

▶ **STEP 3** Contract the erector spinae and quadratus lumborum to extend the lower back. Extending the lower back tilts the pelvis forward. This moves the origins of the hamstrings back and away from their insertions, stretching the muscle. Engage the lower third of the trapezius to draw the shoulders down and away from the neck. Note how this action brings the foot closer to the face. Activate the rhomboids to draw the shoulder blades toward the midline, expanding the front of the chest.

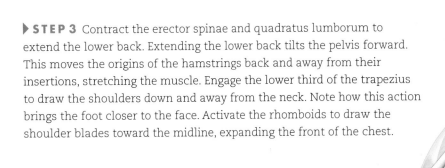

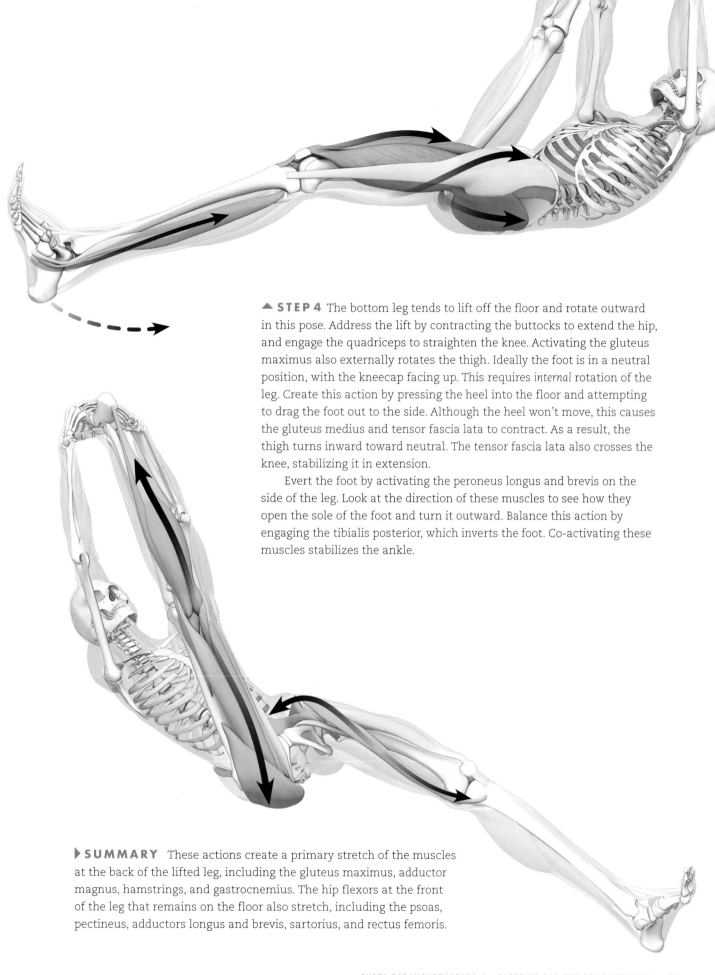

▲ STEP 4 The bottom leg tends to lift off the floor and rotate outward in this pose. Address the lift by contracting the buttocks to extend the hip, and engage the quadriceps to straighten the knee. Activating the gluteus maximus also externally rotates the thigh. Ideally the foot is in a neutral position, with the kneecap facing up. This requires *internal* rotation of the leg. Create this action by pressing the heel into the floor and attempting to drag the foot out to the side. Although the heel won't move, this causes the gluteus medius and tensor fascia lata to contract. As a result, the thigh turns inward toward neutral. The tensor fascia lata also crosses the knee, stabilizing it in extension.

Evert the foot by activating the peroneus longus and brevis on the side of the leg. Look at the direction of these muscles to see how they open the sole of the foot and turn it outward. Balance this action by engaging the tibialis posterior, which inverts the foot. Co-activating these muscles stabilizes the ankle.

▶ SUMMARY These actions create a primary stretch of the muscles at the back of the lifted leg, including the gluteus maximus, adductor magnus, hamstrings, and gastrocnemius. The hip flexors at the front of the leg that remains on the floor also stretch, including the psoas, pectineus, adductors longus and brevis, sartorius, and rectus femoris.

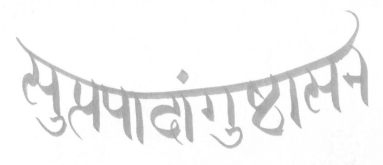

SUPTA PADANGUSTHASANA

SLEEPING BIG-TOE POSE, REVOLVING VERSION

TWO OPPOSING STORIES TAKE PLACE SIMULTANEOUSLY IN THE REVOLVING VARIATION of Supta Padangusthasana. The shoulders and chest turn in one direction, while the pelvis and lower body turn in another. Engage muscles that create this turning to enhance the twist in the pose. Note how drawing the shoulder blade on the free-hand side toward the midline turns the chest away from the pelvis. Similarly, adducting the thigh of the held leg draws the pelvis in an opposite direction to the shoulders. Finally, you can create a bandha by simultaneously pressing down on the foot with the hand and pressing against the hand with the foot. This activates the abductor muscles of the thigh and stabilizes the pelvis once the leg is revolved. Observe how straightening the elbow synergizes the action. Compare this to the cue that we gave in the standing pose Parivrtta Trikonasana, where we pressed the hand against the outer ankle and the foot against the hand. The effect is the same. In fact, one pose can be used to improve the other.

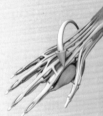

The lower body presents another story. We flex and internally rotate the upper leg while extending the lower leg. The upper leg adducts across the trunk in the opposite direction of the shoulder girdle, thereby rotating the spine. The vertebral column connects the shoulder girdle and pelvis and brings continuity to these two opposing stories. The breath is your soundtrack.

BASIC JOINT POSITIONS

- The hip of the leg on the floor extends and internally rotates.
- The hip of the leg that crosses over the body adducts and internally rotates.
- The knees extend.
- The ankles plantar flex.

- The feet evert.
- The trunk rotates.
- The shoulders abduct and externally rotate.
- The elbows extend.
- The forearms pronate.

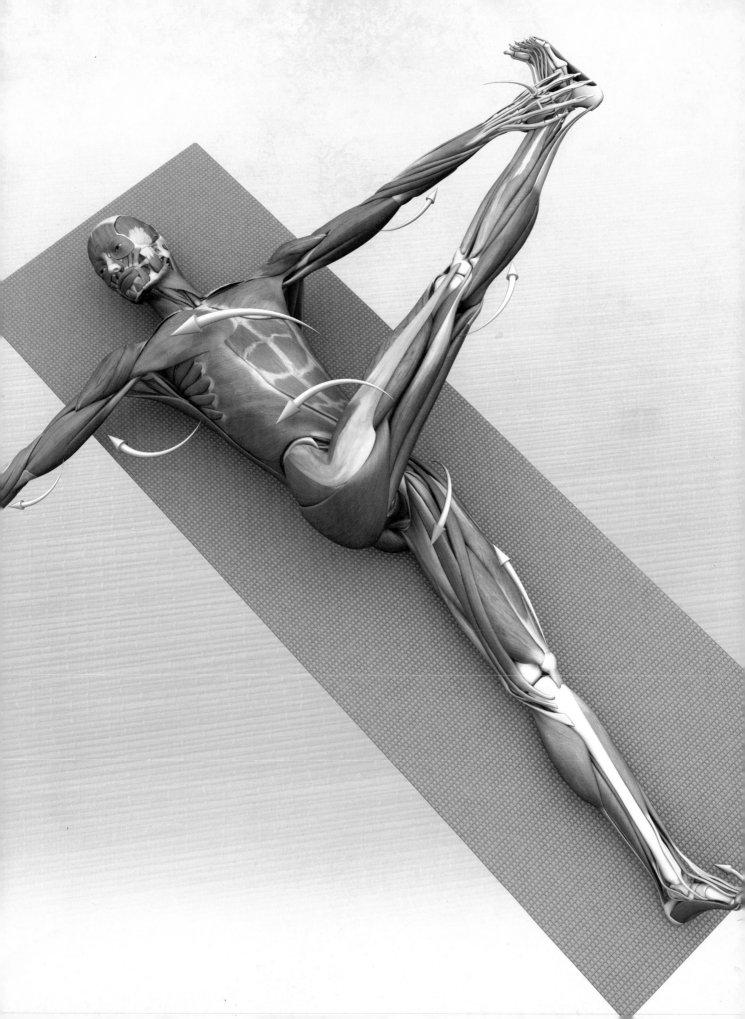

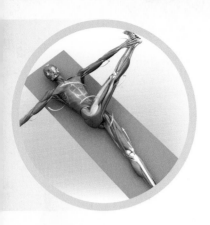

Supta Padangusthasana Preparation

Begin by using a belt to hold the foot, and draw the upper-side leg across the body. Use the opposite-side shoulder and arm to turn the upper body and chest away from the leg. As you gain flexibility, grasp the outer edge of the foot and press down with the palm of the hand to turn the hips. Then straighten and extend the leg that remains on the floor by engaging the buttocks muscles. Brace the body before you ease out of the asana. Use poses such as Marichyasana III to prepare the torso for the twist.

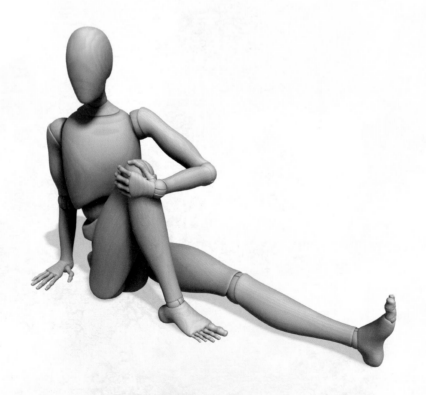

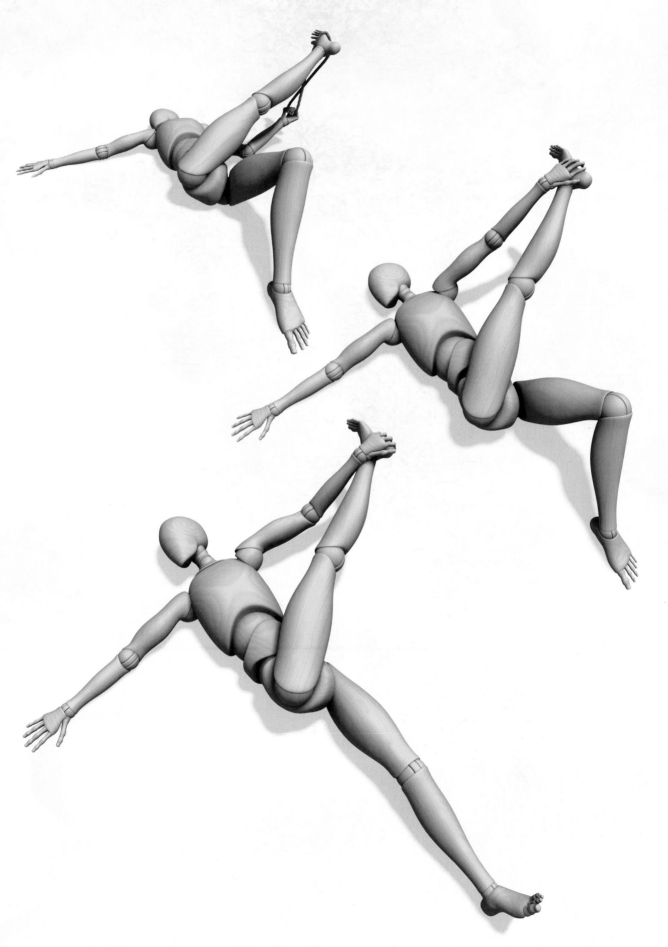

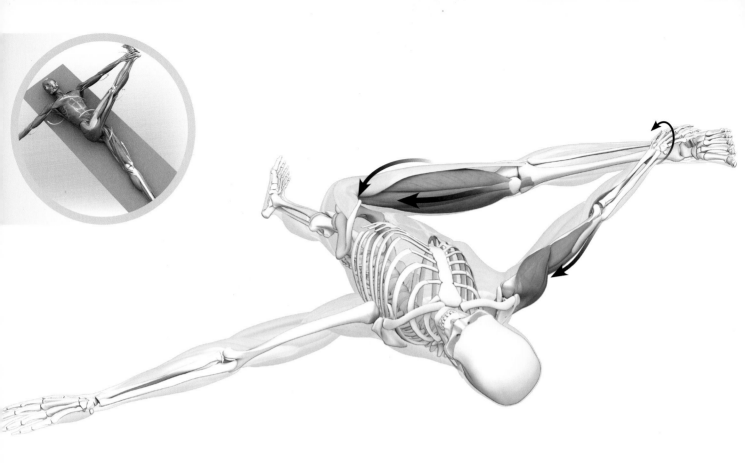

STEP 1 Activate the psoas and its synergists to flex the hip (synergists include the tensor fascia lata, pectineus, adductors longus and brevis, and gluteus minimus). Eccentrically contract the tensor fascia lata to press the side of the leg into the hand—this cue mimics abducting the femur, one action of this muscle; it also stabilizes and internally rotates the femur in the hip joint. Engage the quadriceps to straighten the knee. Extend the elbow and pronate the forearm (turn the palm to face down). Extend the shoulder to press the foot towards the floor, activating the posterior deltoid. Abduct the shoulder to draw the leg upward, contracting the lateral deltoid. This is an example of connecting the upper and lower extremities to dynamize the twist of the torso.

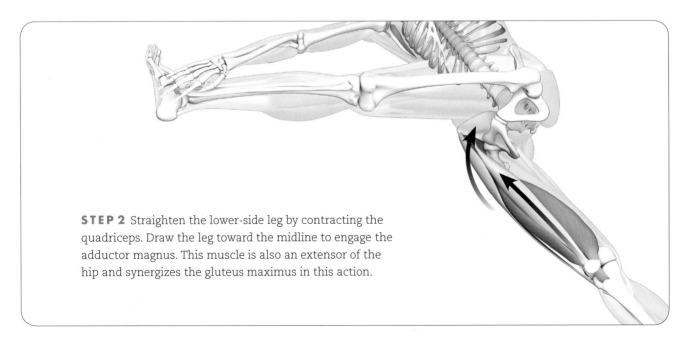

STEP 2 Straighten the lower-side leg by contracting the quadriceps. Draw the leg toward the midline to engage the adductor magnus. This muscle is also an extensor of the hip and synergizes the gluteus maximus in this action.

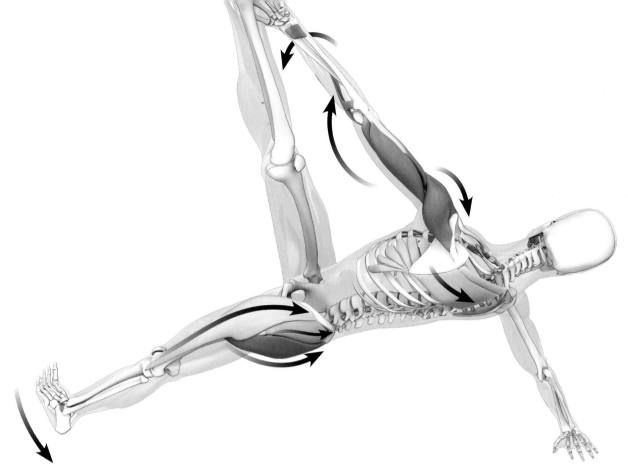

STEP 3 Create opposing actions between the upper and lower body. This image shows the muscles of the arm pressing down onto the foot. Turn the palm down by engaging the pronators teres and quadratus of the forearms. Straighten the elbow with the triceps. Press down onto the foot with the lateral and posterior portions of the deltoid. Draw the shoulder blade toward the midline by engaging the rhomboids.

The serratus anterior expands the chest, drawing the shoulder and arm in the direction of the foot. At the same time, extend the lower-side leg by activating the gluteus maximus. Note that this action has the side effect of turning the foot outward. Oppose this by pressing the heel into the floor and attempting to draw the foot away from the midline. Using this cue engages the tensor fascia lata and internally rotates the femur at the hip, opposing the external rotational force of the gluteus maximus.

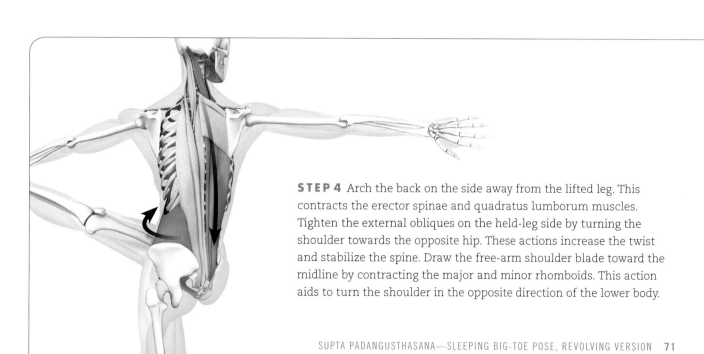

STEP 4 Arch the back on the side away from the lifted leg. This contracts the erector spinae and quadratus lumborum muscles. Tighten the external obliques on the held-leg side by turning the shoulder towards the opposite hip. These actions increase the twist and stabilize the spine. Draw the free-arm shoulder blade toward the midline by contracting the major and minor rhomboids. This action aids to turn the shoulder in the opposite direction of the lower body.

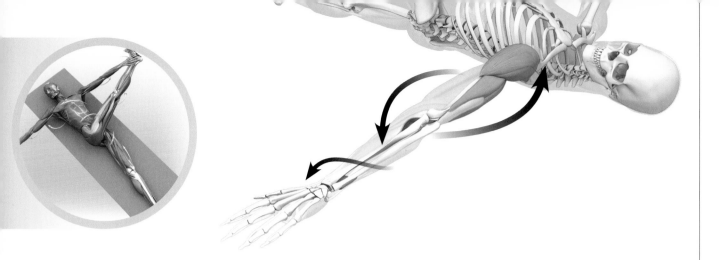

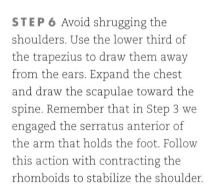

STEP 5 Abduct the shoulder with the lateral deltoid, and draw the hand toward the floor with the posterior deltoid. Contract the triceps. Engage the pronators teres and quadratus of the forearm to turn the palm to face downwards. Connect this with the rhomboids on this side to draw the scapula toward the midline, turning the shoulders and chest away from the pelvis.

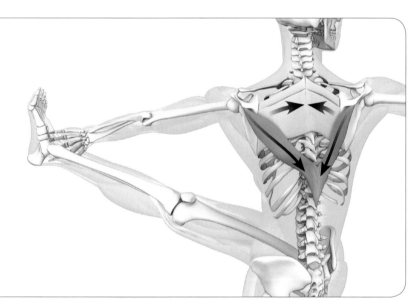

STEP 6 Avoid shrugging the shoulders. Use the lower third of the trapezius to draw them away from the ears. Expand the chest and draw the scapulae toward the spine. Remember that in Step 3 we engaged the serratus anterior of the arm that holds the foot. Follow this action with contracting the rhomboids to stabilize the shoulder.

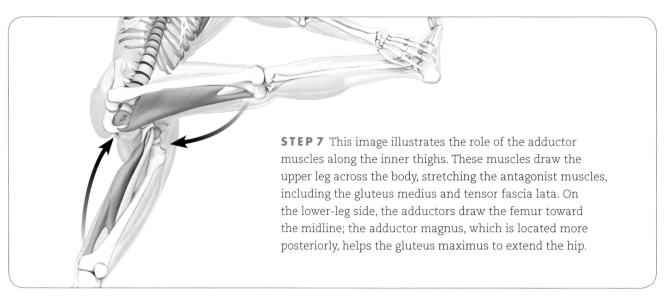

STEP 7 This image illustrates the role of the adductor muscles along the inner thighs. These muscles draw the upper leg across the body, stretching the antagonist muscles, including the gluteus medius and tensor fascia lata. On the lower-leg side, the adductors draw the femur toward the midline; the adductor magnus, which is located more posteriorly, helps the gluteus maximus to extend the hip.

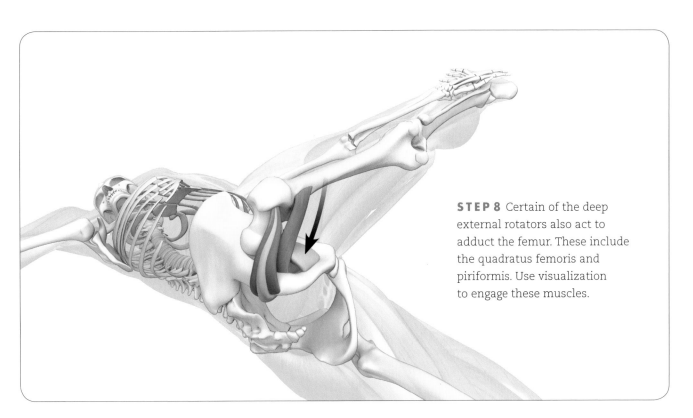

STEP 8 Certain of the deep external rotators also act to adduct the femur. These include the quadratus femoris and piriformis. Use visualization to engage these muscles.

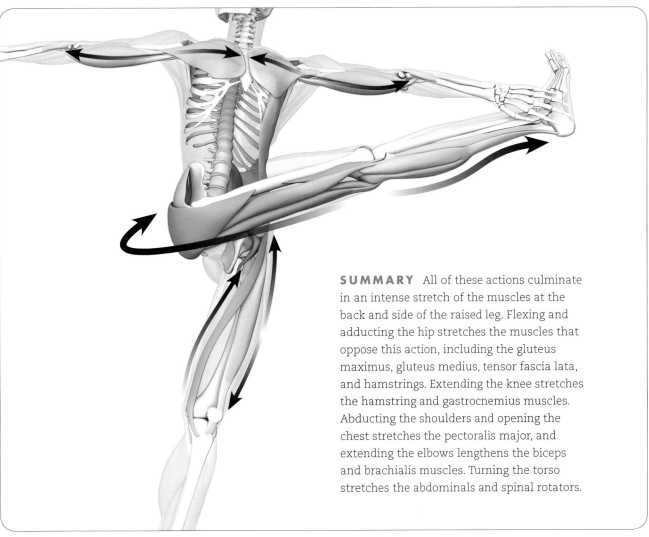

SUMMARY All of these actions culminate in an intense stretch of the muscles at the back and side of the raised leg. Flexing and adducting the hip stretches the muscles that oppose this action, including the gluteus maximus, gluteus medius, tensor fascia lata, and hamstrings. Extending the knee stretches the hamstring and gastrocnemius muscles. Abducting the shoulders and opening the chest stretches the pectoralis major, and extending the elbows lengthens the biceps and brachialis muscles. Turning the torso stretches the abdominals and spinal rotators.

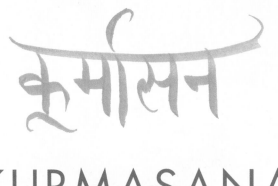

KURMASANA

TORTOISE POSE

THE ANCIENT YOGIS CREATED AN INGENIOUS SOLUTION TO STRETCHING hard-to-access muscles—Kurmasana. In this pose we connect the arms and legs to stretch the lower back and hips. The main story here is the trunk flexing forward. Linking the elbows behind the knees creates a subplot to this story. You can see that straightening the knees presses down on the backs of the arms and flexes the trunk deeper. Contract the biceps and brachialis muscles to bend the elbows and protect them from hyperextending. When the thighs press onto the upper arms, attempting to bend the elbows with the palms fixed on the floor draws the torso deeper into the pose, giving that extra inch or two of stretch where yoga really happens.

BASIC JOINT POSITIONS

- The hips flex and abduct.
- The knees extend.
- The ankles plantar flex.
- The feet evert.
- The trunk flexes.

- The shoulders extend, abduct, and externally rotate.
- The elbows extend.
- The forearms pronate.

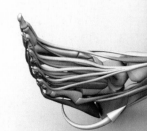

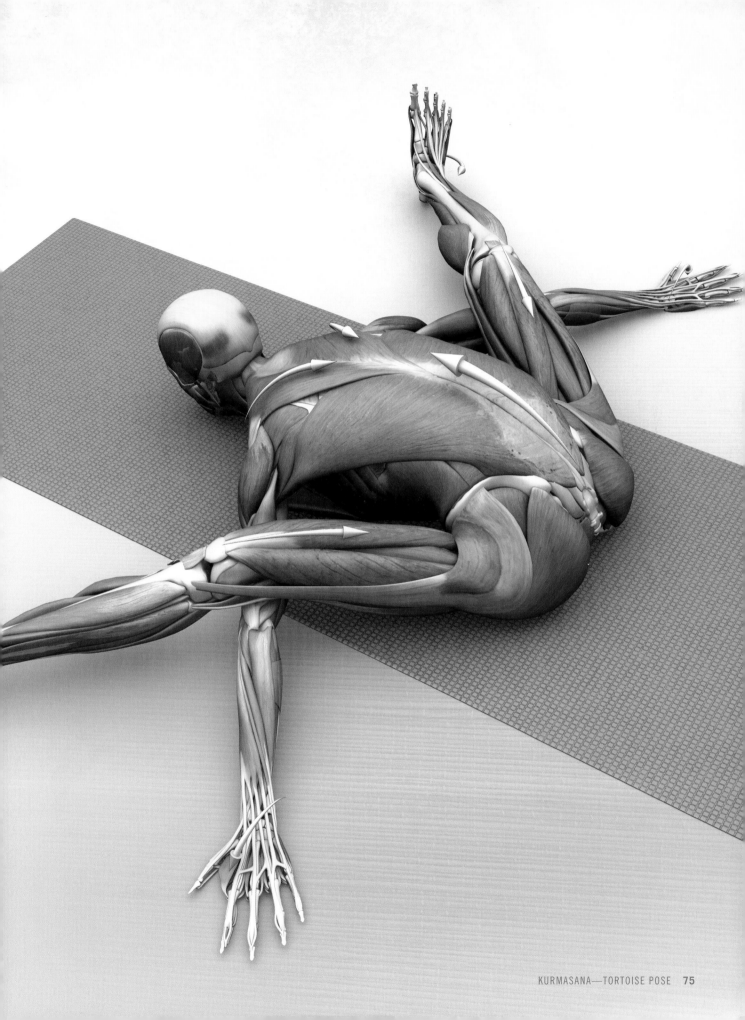

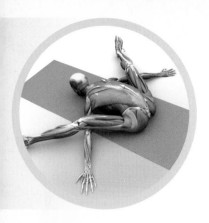

Kurmasana Preparation

Get a feeling for the stretch by starting with the knees and elbows bent. This may be as far as you will want to go in the pose. Then gently press the backs of the knees into the upper arms, keeping the elbows bent to protect them from hyper-extending. As you become more flexible, move the thighs higher up on the backs of the arms, above the elbows, to gain greater leverage in pressing the trunk down when you straighten the knees. Use poses such as the bent-knee version of Supta Padangusthasana to prepare the gluteals and upper portion of the hamstrings and Upavistha Konasana to stretch the back muscles.

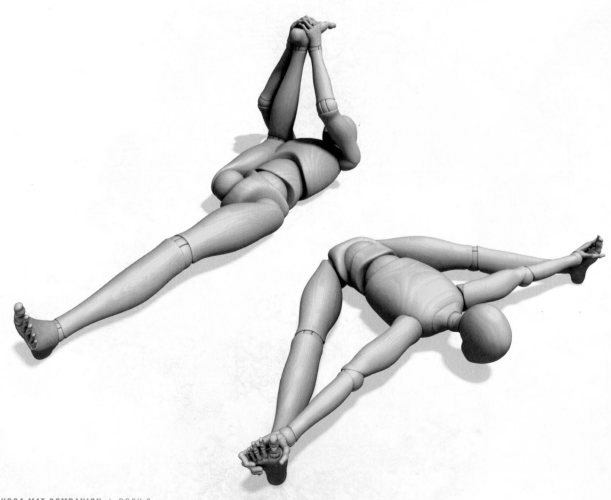

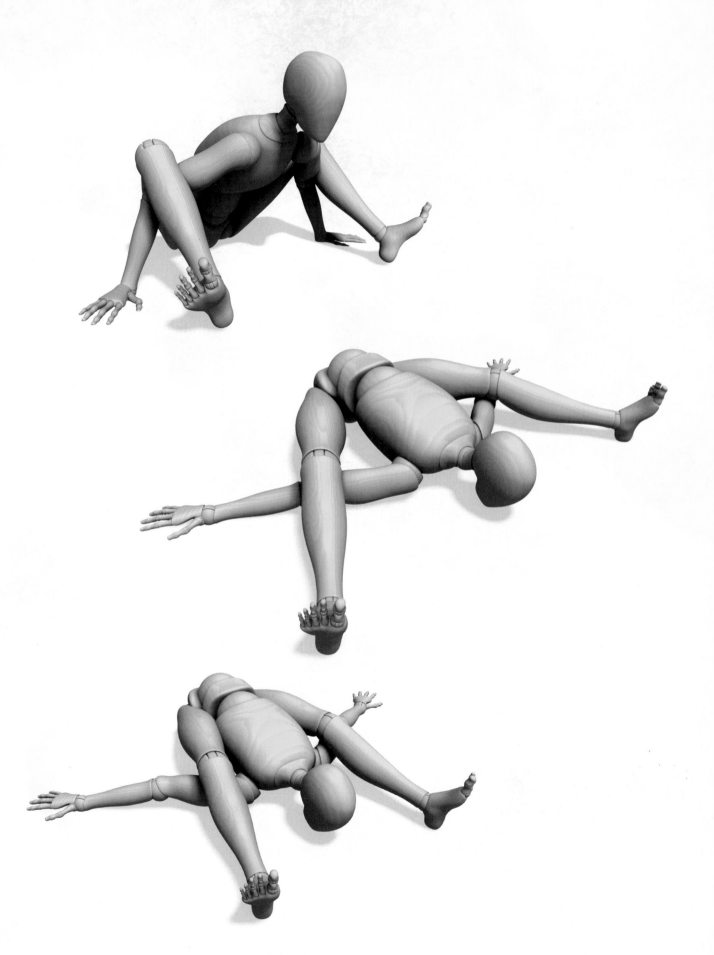

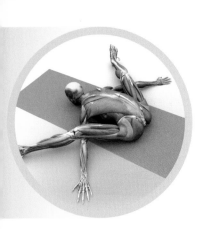

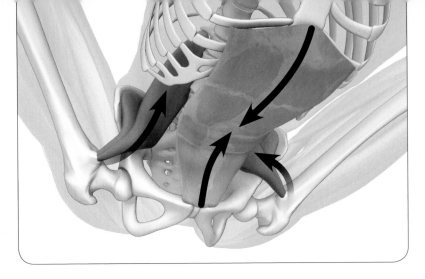

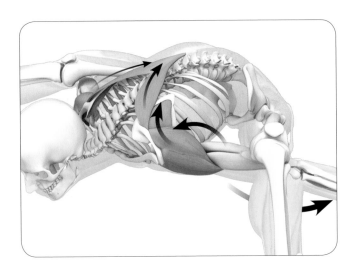

STEP 1 Contract the abdominals to flex the trunk. Activate the psoas to flex the femurs. The psoas major originates from the lumbar spine and, as such, aids to draw the trunk deeper into the pose. Be aware, however, that the hips are fully flexed and that the hip flexors have limited capacity to contract further and add to this movement. In situations like this, you can connect the upper and lower extremities to deepen the pose.

STEP 2 Place the arms under the legs with the palms on the floor. Press the mounds at the base of the index fingers down to pronate the forearms, using the pronator teres and quadratus muscles. As you enter the pose, extend the elbows by contracting the triceps to deepen the placement of the arms under the legs. Attempt to lift the elbows and upper arm bones against the backs of the legs. This engages the lateral and posterior portions of the deltoids, flexing the trunk deeper. Draw the shoulders away from the ears by contracting the lower third of the trapezius.

STEP 3 Straighten the knees by activating the quadriceps. This presses the legs onto the backs of the arms and creates an intense stretch of the back muscles and of the gluteus maximus, the main hip extensor. The pull of the stretching gluteus draws the thighs into external rotation, turning the kneecaps outward. Use the tensor fascia lata to counteract this by rotating the femurs inward. The cue for this is to press the heels into the mat and attempt to drag the feet apart. The feet will not move because they are constrained on the mat, but the tensor fascia lata and gluteus medius will contract and internally rotate the femurs. If you look under the tensor fascia lata here, you will see the gluteus minimus. This muscle synergizes hip flexion and internal rotation and stabilizes the head of the femur in the socket. Visualize it in action when practicing Kurmasana.

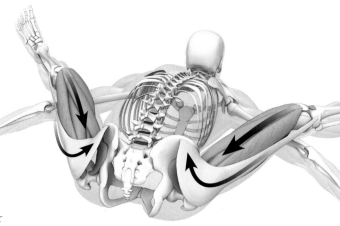

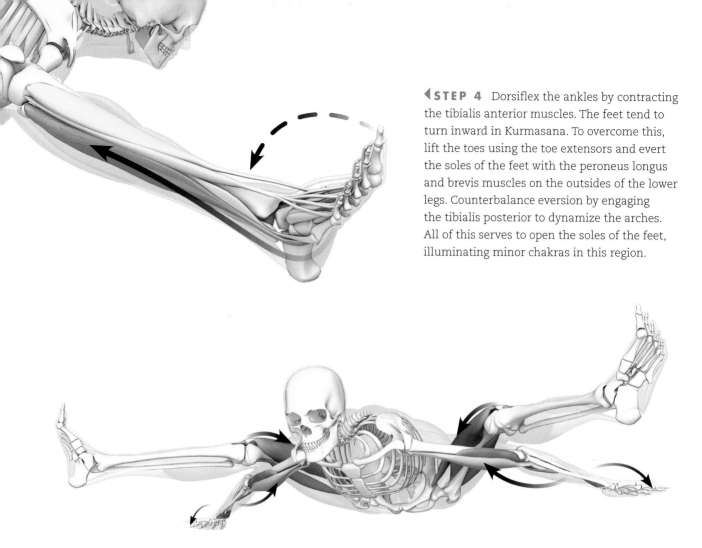

◀ **STEP 4** Dorsiflex the ankles by contracting the tibialis anterior muscles. The feet tend to turn inward in Kurmasana. To overcome this, lift the toes using the toe extensors and evert the soles of the feet with the peroneus longus and brevis muscles on the outsides of the lower legs. Counterbalance eversion by engaging the tibialis posterior to dynamize the arches. All of this serves to open the soles of the feet, illuminating minor chakras in this region.

▲ **STEP 5** Pronate the forearms with the pronators teres and quadratus. Engage the flexors carpi radialis and ulnaris to flex the wrists. Attempt to bend the elbows by contracting the biceps and brachialis muscles. This protects them against hyperextension and deepens the pose via closed chain contraction of the biceps. Engage the quadriceps to straighten the knees and press the thighs into the backs of the arms, flexing the trunk further. This illustrates how to produce additional movement in the hips and pelvis by connecting the arms and legs.

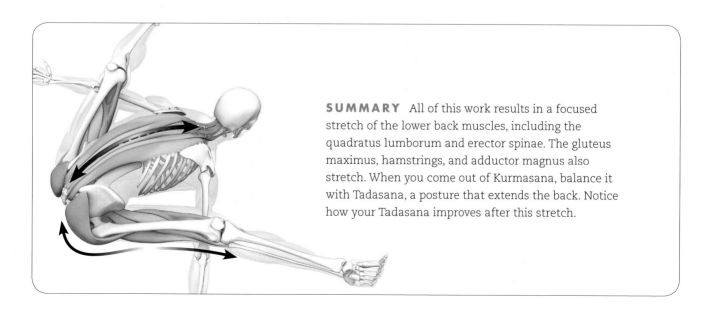

SUMMARY All of this work results in a focused stretch of the lower back muscles, including the quadratus lumborum and erector spinae. The gluteus maximus, hamstrings, and adductor magnus also stretch. When you come out of Kurmasana, balance it with Tadasana, a posture that extends the back. Notice how your Tadasana improves after this stretch.

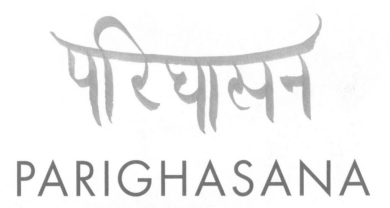

PARIGHASANA

CROSS BAR OF THE GATE POSE

LOOK CLOSELY AND YOU CAN SEE THAT THERE ARE SEVERAL OVERLAPPING STORIES in Parighasana. First, it is a side bend that flexes the trunk over the leg. Second, it is a hip opener that stretches the muscles at the front of the bent-leg pelvis. Balancing along a line between the straight and bent legs also teaches poise. Refine equilibrium by pressing the top of the bent-leg foot and the sole of the straight-leg foot into the mat.

Remember that stability originates from the pelvic core, with the gluteals engaging on one side and the psoas contracting on the other. This produces a bandha across the pelvis, tightening the sacroiliac ligaments to create a "wringing" effect (known as ligamentotaxis) that grounds the pose.

Engage the straight-leg quadriceps to extend the knee and the calf muscles to press the sole of the foot into the mat. Similarly, activate the bent-leg side quadriceps and tibialis anterior to press the top of the foot into the floor. Actively pressing the feet into the floor creates a strong foundation, which connects the bones of the legs to the pelvis, stabilizing it.

BASIC JOINT POSITIONS

- The straight-leg hip flexes and externally rotates.
- The knee extends.
- The ankle plantar flexes.
- The bent-leg hip extends and externally rotates.
- The bent-leg knee flexes.

- The ankles plantar flex.
- The trunk laterally flexes.
- The shoulders flex, abduct, and externally rotate.
- The elbows extend.
- The forearms pronate.

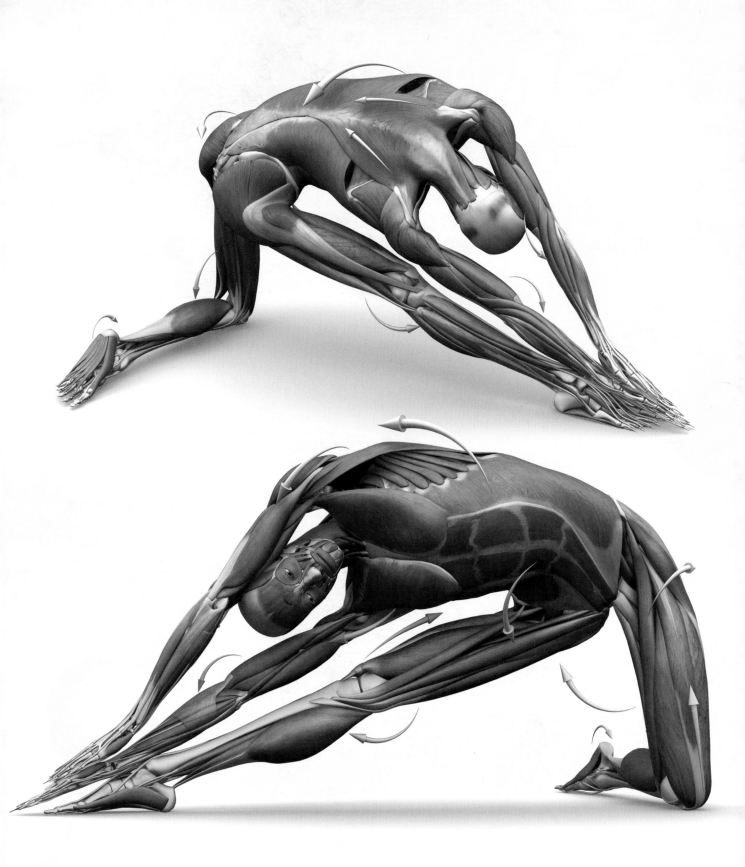

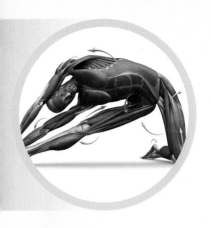

Parighasana Preparation

Use a side bend to stretch the spinal rotators and oblique abdominals; this helps to prepare the muscles of the torso. Another pose that can be used for this is Parighasana I with a belt, which also stretches the side body.

Place the feet as shown, and raise the arms to open the chest; this aids with balance. Then activate the hip flexors to draw the torso over the straight leg, leaning into the pose. Remember to breathe. Brace the body to prepare to come up by firming the upper-side abdominals and bent-leg side gluteals. Carefully come out of the pose.

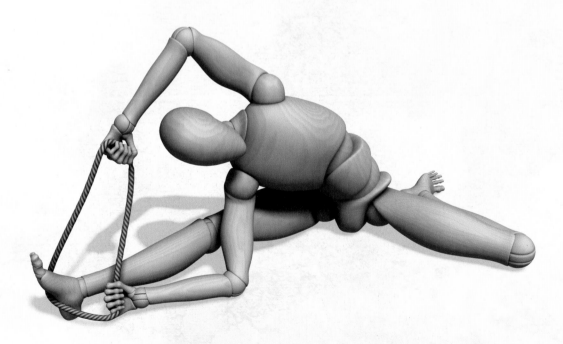

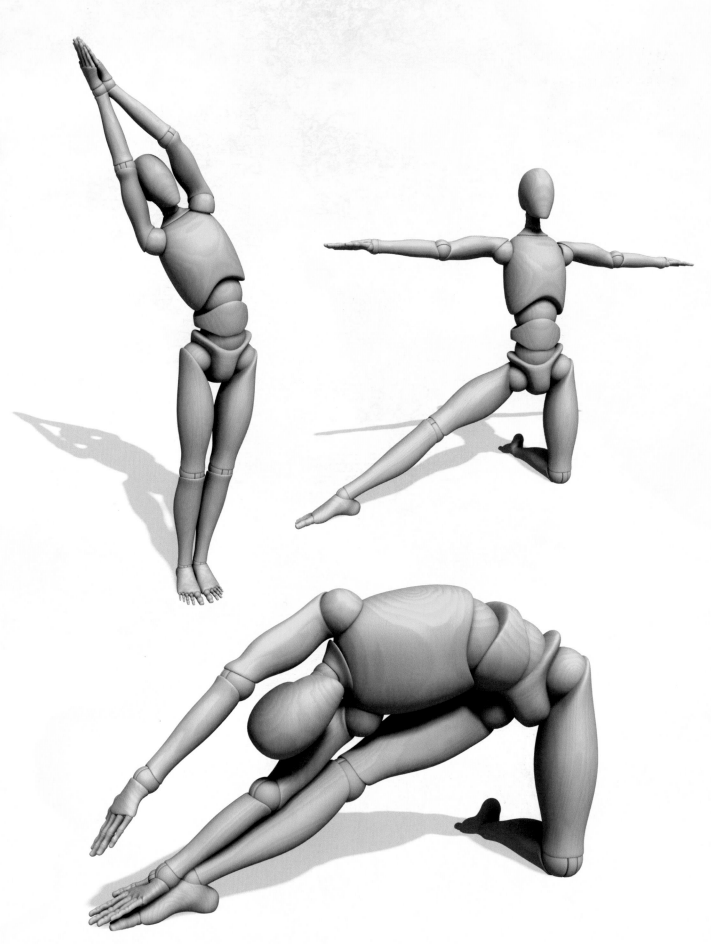

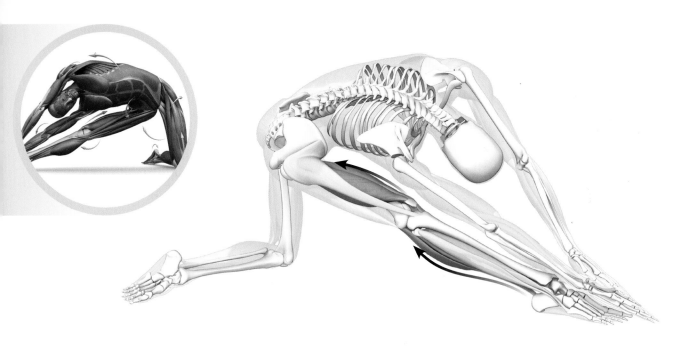

STEP 1 Engage the quadriceps to straighten the knee. A cue for emphasizing this action is to lift the kneecap toward the pelvis. The tensor fascia lata aids to extend the knee and stabilizes it. Press the sole of the foot into the mat by contracting the gastrocnemius and soleus muscles. If the sole won't go flat on the floor, slightly bend the knee, place the foot on the mat, and hold it there by pressing the ball of the foot down. This engages the calf muscles. Then contract the quadriceps to straighten the leg.

Activating the gastrocnemius and soleus muscles plantar flexes the foot and produces reciprocal inhibition of the tibialis anterior at the front of the lower leg, allowing it to lengthen into the stretch. Press the ball of the foot into the mat and spread the weight evenly across the sole by engaging the peroneus longus and brevis muscles. Balance this action with a gentle inversion force at the ankle by contracting the tibialis posterior. These actions combine to lift the arch of the foot.

STEP 2 Gently engage the bent-leg quadriceps to press the top of the shin into the mat. Because the rectus femoris portion of the quadriceps crosses the hip, contracting it connects the front of the lower leg to the pelvis, stabilizing it. Next, squeeze the buttocks to activate the gluteus maximus, extending the hip and lengthening the structures at the front of the pelvis. Plantar flex the ankle by contracting the gastrocnemius and soleus to point the toes and stretch the muscles at the front of the lower leg, including the tibialis anterior and toe extensors. Balance this with eccentric contraction of the tibialis anterior by pressing the top of the foot into the mat.

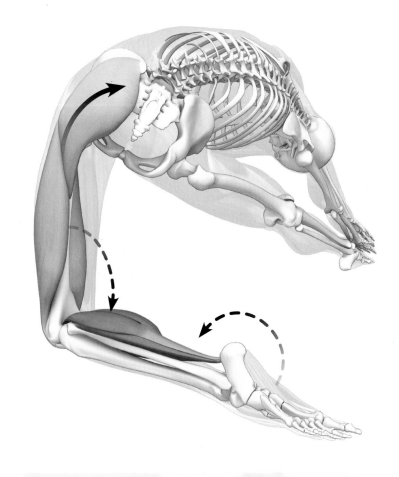

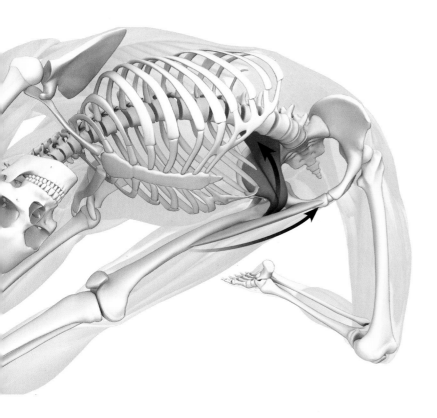

STEP 3 Flex the hip by contracting the psoas and its synergists, the pectineus and sartorius. The tensor fascia lata along with the rectus femoris synergizes this action. The psoas not only flexes the hip, but also tilts the pelvis slightly forward, drawing the lumbar spine towards the leg.

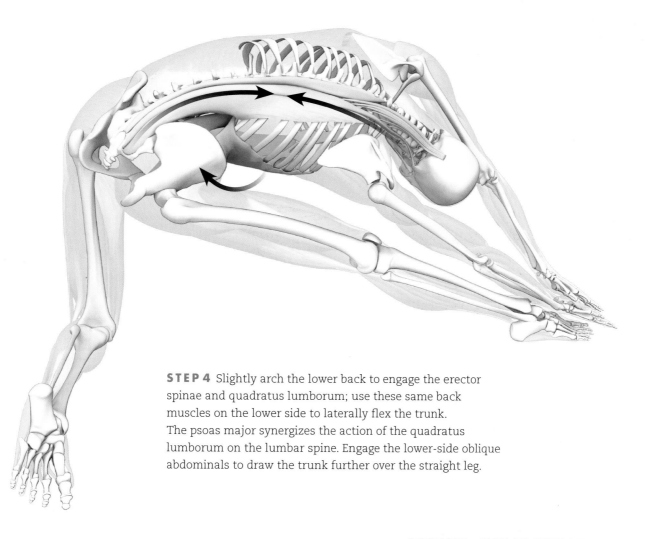

STEP 4 Slightly arch the lower back to engage the erector spinae and quadratus lumborum; use these same back muscles on the lower side to laterally flex the trunk. The psoas major synergizes the action of the quadratus lumborum on the lumbar spine. Engage the lower-side oblique abdominals to draw the trunk further over the straight leg.

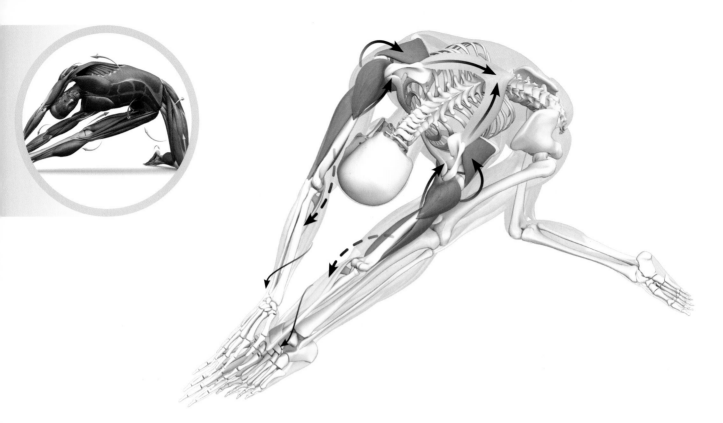

STEP 5 Straighten the arms by activating the triceps. Engage the anterior and lateral portions of the deltoids to lift the upper arm bones (the humeri) over the head. This is forward flexion of the shoulders. Externally rotate the shoulders with the posterior deltoids and the infraspinatus and teres minor muscles. Then draw the scapulae away from the neck by activating the lower third of the trapezius.

Finally, add the pronators teres and quadratus to create a "coiling" effect up and down the arms. The cue for this action is to press the mounds at the base of the index fingers together. Note how this rotates the forearms in the opposite direction of the shoulders (which externally rotate), producing ligamentotaxis through the elbows.

STEP 6 Attempt to drag the bent-leg knee toward the foot of the extended leg on the mat. The knee will not actually move because it is constrained on the mat; however, this cue activates the adductors on the bent-leg side and the hamstrings on the straight-leg side. Balance these forces to draw the energy up into the pelvis.

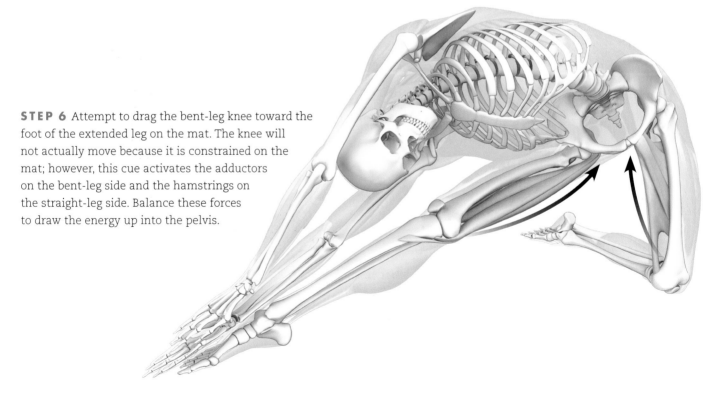

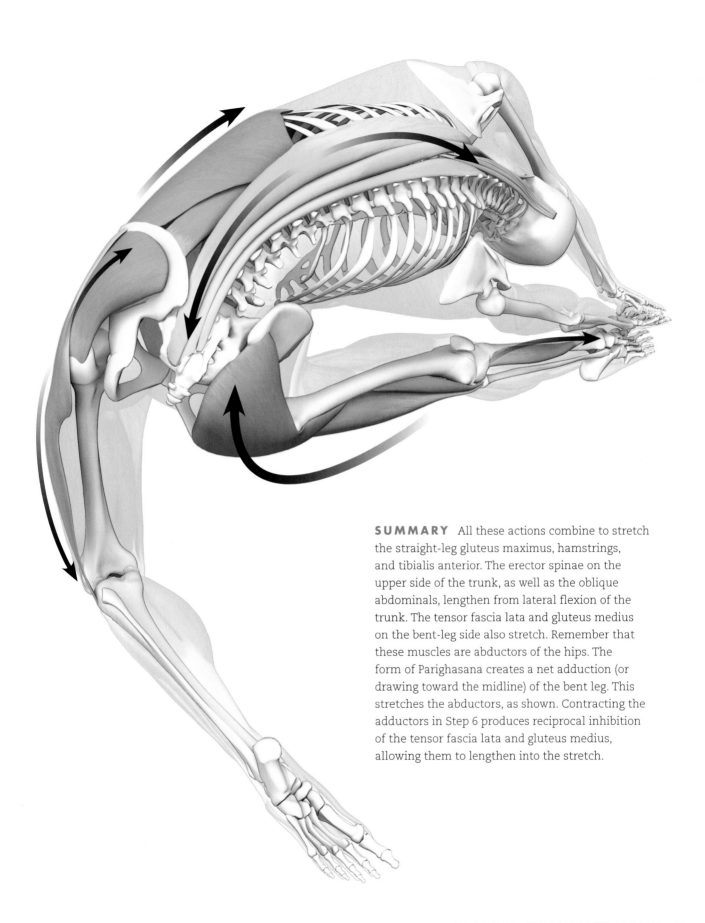

SUMMARY All these actions combine to stretch the straight-leg gluteus maximus, hamstrings, and tibialis anterior. The erector spinae on the upper side of the trunk, as well as the oblique abdominals, lengthen from lateral flexion of the trunk. The tensor fascia lata and gluteus medius on the bent-leg side also stretch. Remember that these muscles are abductors of the hips. The form of Parighasana creates a net adduction (or drawing toward the midline) of the bent leg. This stretches the abductors, as shown. Contracting the adductors in Step 6 produces reciprocal inhibition of the tensor fascia lata and gluteus medius, allowing them to lengthen into the stretch.

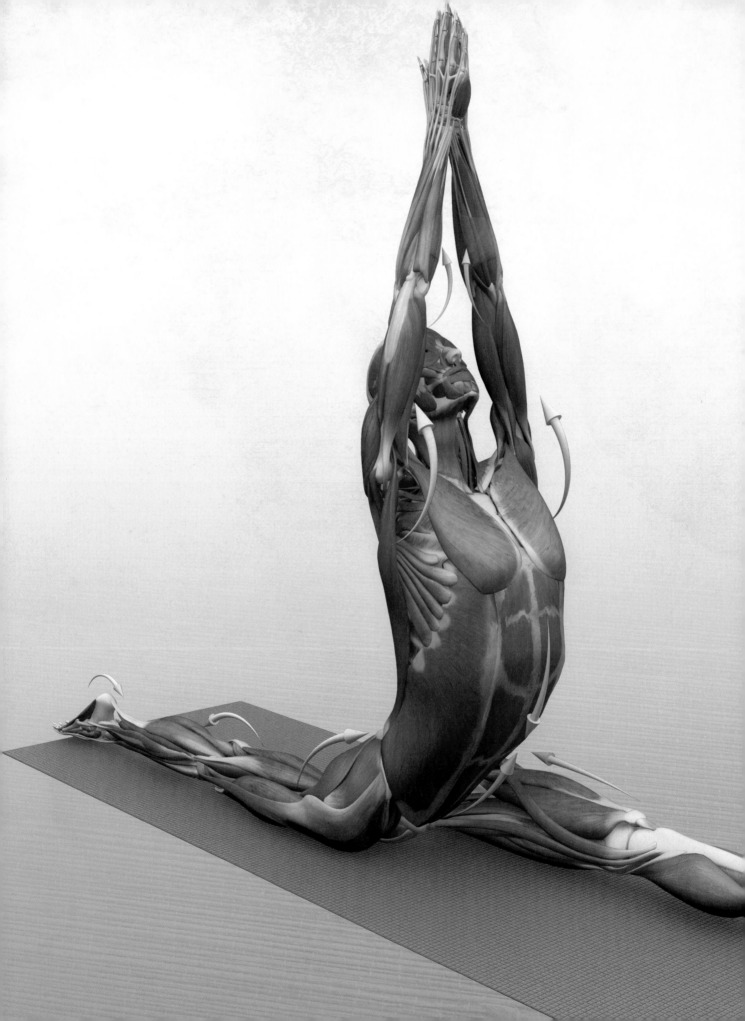

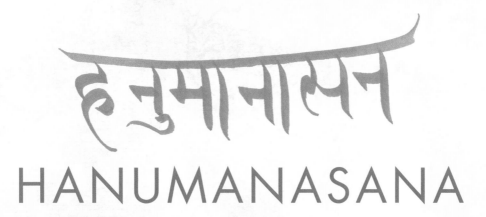

HANUMANASANA

MONKEY POSE

IN HANUMANASANA, THE BODY PROJECTS IN FOUR DIRECTIONS simultaneously—forward and back, upward and down. The story of Hanuman, the Monkey God, is that he bridged two worlds between his feet to save the wife of Rama (an ancient king of India). The wide spread of the legs represents a tribute to the Monkey God's great leap across the worlds. The back leg is the constraining force holding the body to the earth, and the front leg reaches forward into the other world. The back hip extends, adducts, and internally rotates. The front hip flexes, and the knee extends the leg forward. As in Pigeon Pose, engaging the extensors of the back hip and the flexors of the front hip creates a "wringing" force across the ligaments of the pelvis, stabilizing and anchoring it to the floor. The back extends and the chest opens upward with the help of the shoulders and arms.

BASIC JOINT POSITIONS

- The forward-leg hip flexes.
- The rear-leg hip extends.
- The knees extend.
- The ankles plantar flex.

- The trunk extends.
- The shoulders flex, abduct, and externally rotate.
- The elbows extend.
- The forearms pronate.

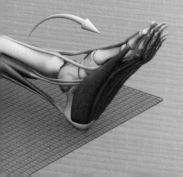

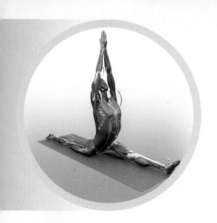

Hanumanasana Preparation

Use a chair to support the upper body and take the general form of the pose by extending the back hip and flexing the front hip. Contract the hip extensors by squeezing the buttocks of the back leg. Engage the hip flexors by attempting to lift the front leg. Keep the knees slightly bent in the beginning. Gradually allow the body to deepen into the pose. Engaging the muscles that produce this form creates a sensory image of the pose in the brain. See additional instructions on how to use facilitated stretching to obtain Hanumanasana on page 14.

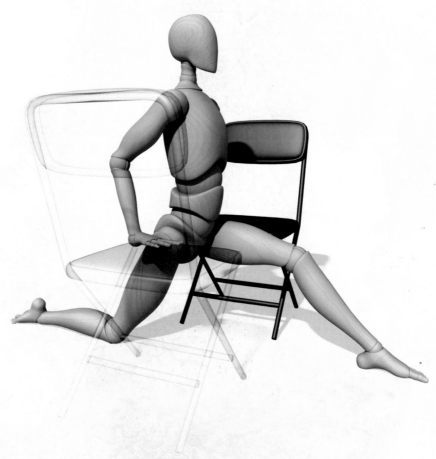

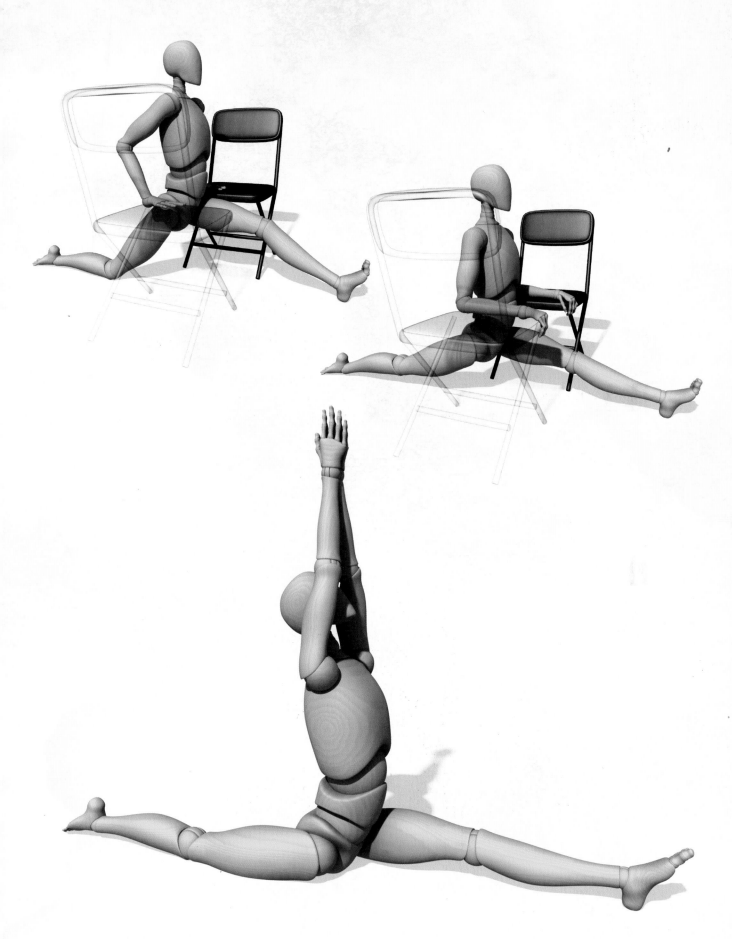

HANUMANASANA—MONKEY POSE 91

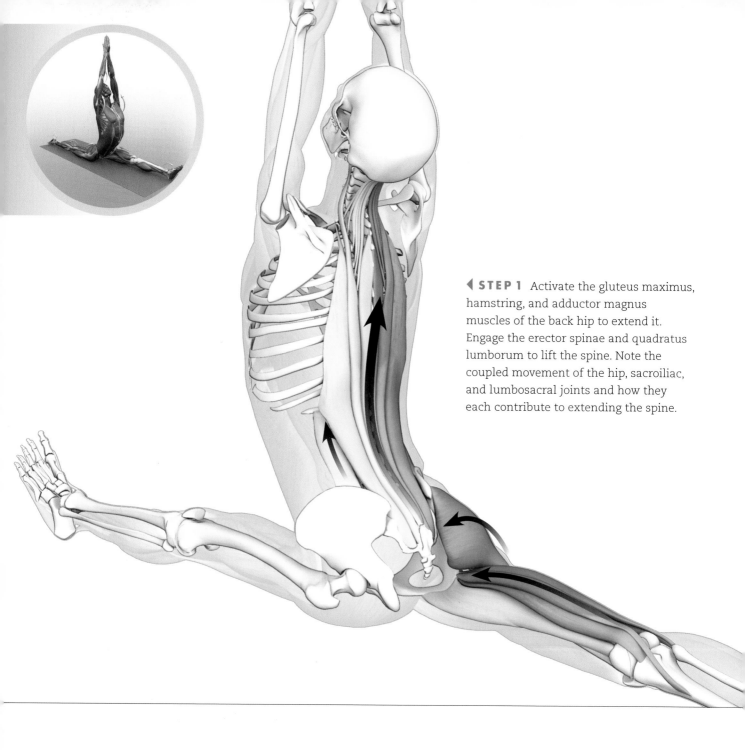

◀ STEP 1 Activate the gluteus maximus, hamstring, and adductor magnus muscles of the back hip to extend it. Engage the erector spinae and quadratus lumborum to lift the spine. Note the coupled movement of the hip, sacroiliac, and lumbosacral joints and how they each contribute to extending the spine.

STEP 2 ▶▶ The back leg tends to roll outward in Hanumanasana due to the external rotation component of the gluteus maximus. Counteract this by contracting the gluteus medius and tensor fascia lata. The cue for this is to press the top of the foot into the mat and attempt to drag it out to the side. The foot won't actually move, but engaging these muscles will internally rotate the hip and leg.

Activate the quadriceps to straighten the back knee. One of the quadriceps, the rectus femoris, crosses the hip and tilts the pelvis forward (anteversion). This action synergizes with the psoas on the other hip, which wraps over the front of the pelvis and also tilts it forward. Anteverting the pelvis releases the anterior iliofemoral ligament (also known as the "anti-Hanuman ligament" because it can block

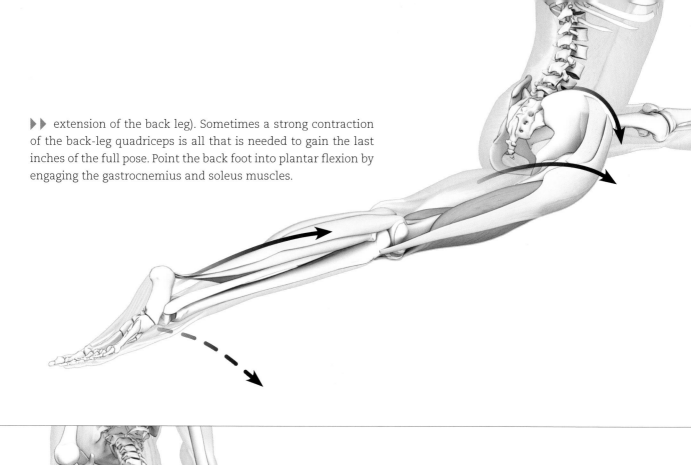

▶▶ extension of the back leg). Sometimes a strong contraction of the back-leg quadriceps is all that is needed to gain the last inches of the full pose. Point the back foot into plantar flexion by engaging the gastrocnemius and soleus muscles.

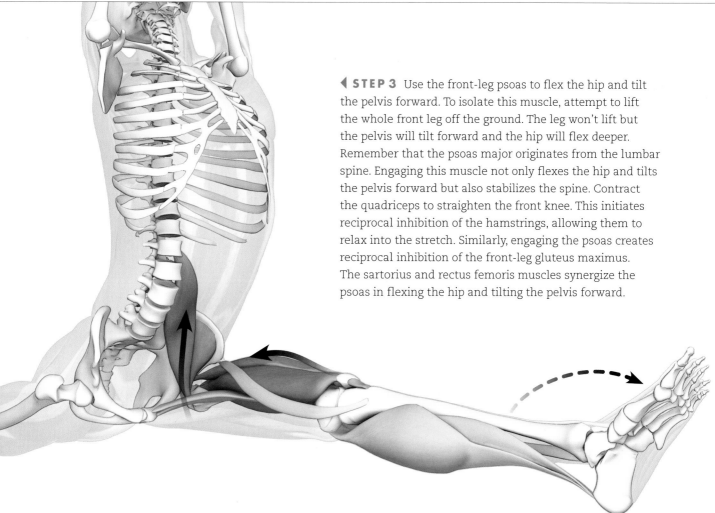

◀ **STEP 3** Use the front-leg psoas to flex the hip and tilt the pelvis forward. To isolate this muscle, attempt to lift the whole front leg off the ground. The leg won't lift but the pelvis will tilt forward and the hip will flex deeper. Remember that the psoas major originates from the lumbar spine. Engaging this muscle not only flexes the hip and tilts the pelvis forward but also stabilizes the spine. Contract the quadriceps to straighten the front knee. This initiates reciprocal inhibition of the hamstrings, allowing them to relax into the stretch. Similarly, engaging the psoas creates reciprocal inhibition of the front-leg gluteus maximus. The sartorius and rectus femoris muscles synergize the psoas in flexing the hip and tilting the pelvis forward.

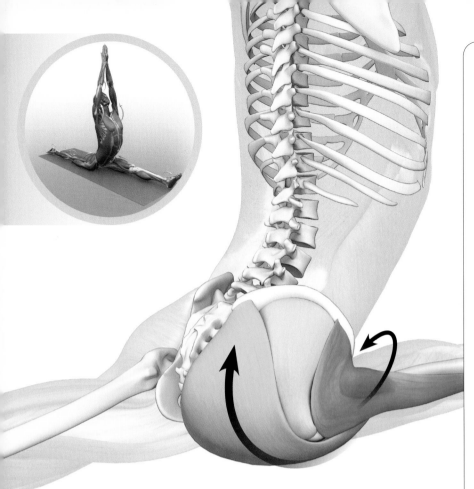

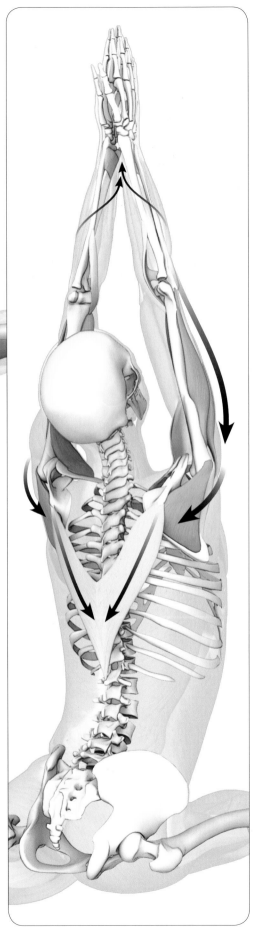

▲ **STEP 4** The front-leg gluteus maximus stretches in this pose and tends to pull on the femur, rotating it outward. Activate the tensor fascia lata to counteract this external rotation and bring the kneecap to face straight up. A cue for this is to press the front-leg heel into the mat and attempt to drag it out to the side. The heel won't move because it is constrained to the mat, but the action engages the internal rotation component of the tensor fascia lata, turning the thigh inward.

▶ **STEP 5** Raise the arms by engaging the anterior deltoids. Externally rotate the shoulders by contracting the infraspinatus and teres minor muscles, and engage the triceps to extend the elbows. Note that the long head of the triceps attaches to the scapula. You can activate this muscle to rotate the scapula outward. This draws the acromion process away from the humerus, allowing the arm to rise higher up and further back. Get a feel for this action by attempting to lift the arms straight up in front of you without strongly contracting the triceps. You will notice that the shoulders meet with a point of resistance that prevents further movement. Then strongly engage the triceps and note how you can gain an extra inch or so of backward movement when you raise the arms.

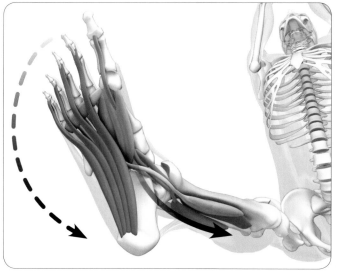

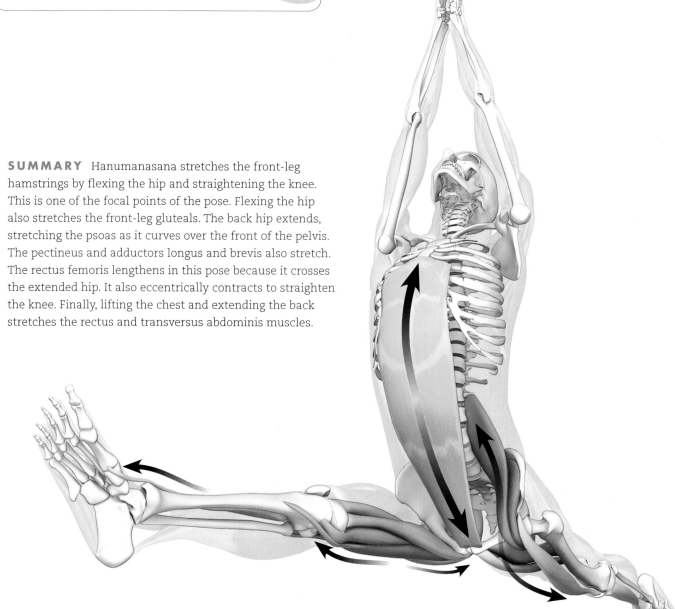

◀ STEP 6 Contract the gastrocnemius/soleus complex (not pictured) to plantar flex the front ankle. Engage the peroneus longus and brevis muscles to evert the ankle. Create an inversion counterforce to this action by activating the tibialis posterior. Note how this stabilizes the ankle and dynamizes the arch of the foot.

SUMMARY Hanumanasana stretches the front-leg hamstrings by flexing the hip and straightening the knee. This is one of the focal points of the pose. Flexing the hip also stretches the front-leg gluteals. The back hip extends, stretching the psoas as it curves over the front of the pelvis. The pectineus and adductors longus and brevis also stretch. The rectus femoris lengthens in this pose because it crosses the extended hip. It also eccentrically contracts to straighten the knee. Finally, lifting the chest and extending the back stretches the rectus and transversus abdominis muscles.

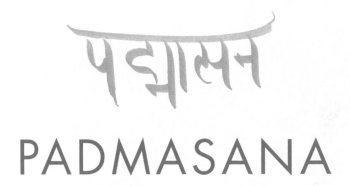

PADMASANA

LOTUS POSE

LOTUS POSE IS ONE OF THE MOST ADVANCED OF THE HIP-OPENING ASANAS. It is a continuation of Sukhasana (Easy Cross-Legged Pose), with the hips flexing, abducting, and externally rotating. The feet are brought up onto the thighs and a bandha is formed where the lower legs cross.

Achieving Lotus safely requires great flexibility in the hips—especially in external rotation. This means that the muscles that *internally* rotate the hips must be brought out to full length. Conversely, if Padmasana is attempted with tight internal rotators, the knees can be injured because the rotational forces of the pose are transmitted to the knee, which should be maintained as a hinge. The hip, on the other hand, is a ball and socket joint that is designed to rotate. Therefore, we must lengthen the tensor fascia lata and gluteus medius muscles (the internal rotators) to take the rotational forces of this pose into the hips.

Never force the feet into Lotus position as this can injure the knees. Take as long as necessary to gain the required flexibility first.

BASIC JOINT POSITIONS

- The hips flex, abduct, and externally rotate.
- The knees flex.
- The ankles plantar flex.
- The feet evert.

- The trunk extends.
- The shoulders flex and externally rotate.
- The elbows flex.

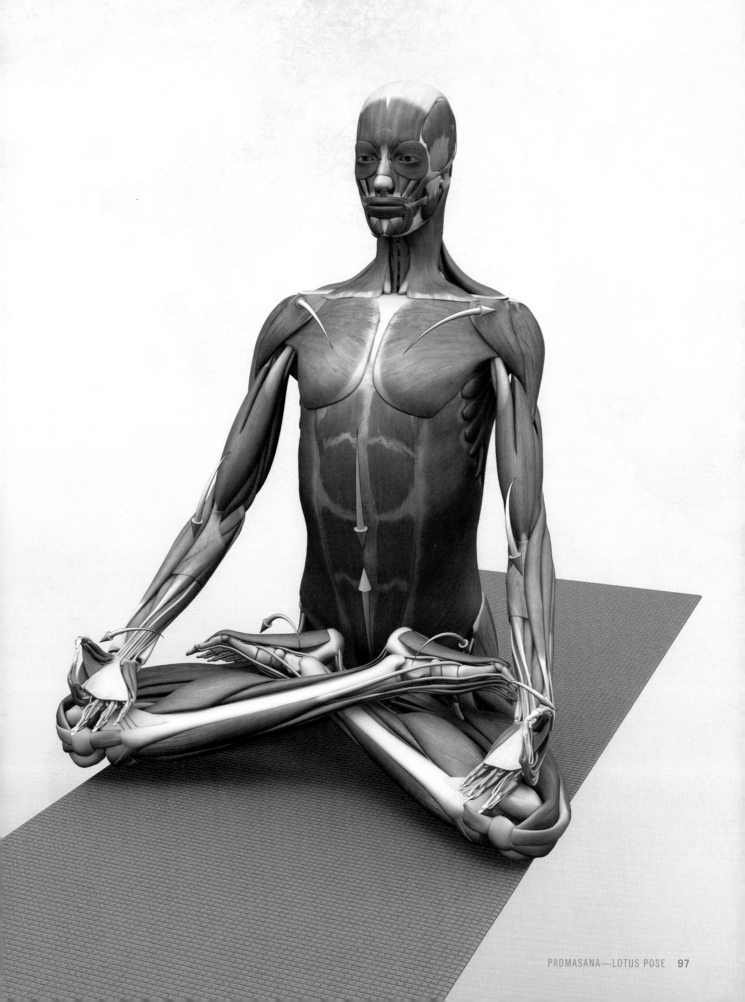

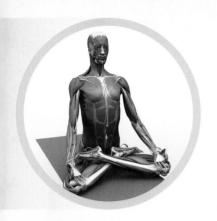

Padmasana Preparation

Lengthen the internal hip rotators using a facilitated stretch, as shown. Cradle the lower leg in the arms while protecting the knee joint by supporting it with the forearm and elbow. Do this stretch on both sides and then place one foot into Half-Lotus (Ardha Padmasana) position. Rest there, and then come out of the pose; take Dandasana to stretch out the knees. Add Ardha Matsyendrasana as a variation to further lengthen the internal rotators.

When both hips have sufficient flexibility, gently place the other foot on top of the leg as shown, hooking the tops of the feet onto the upper thighs. Brace the knees to come out of the asana and straighten the legs again in Dandasana.

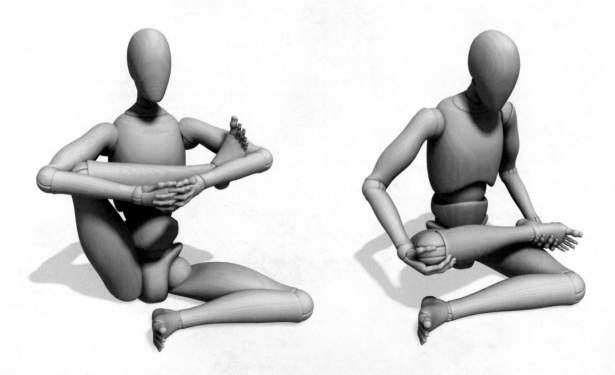

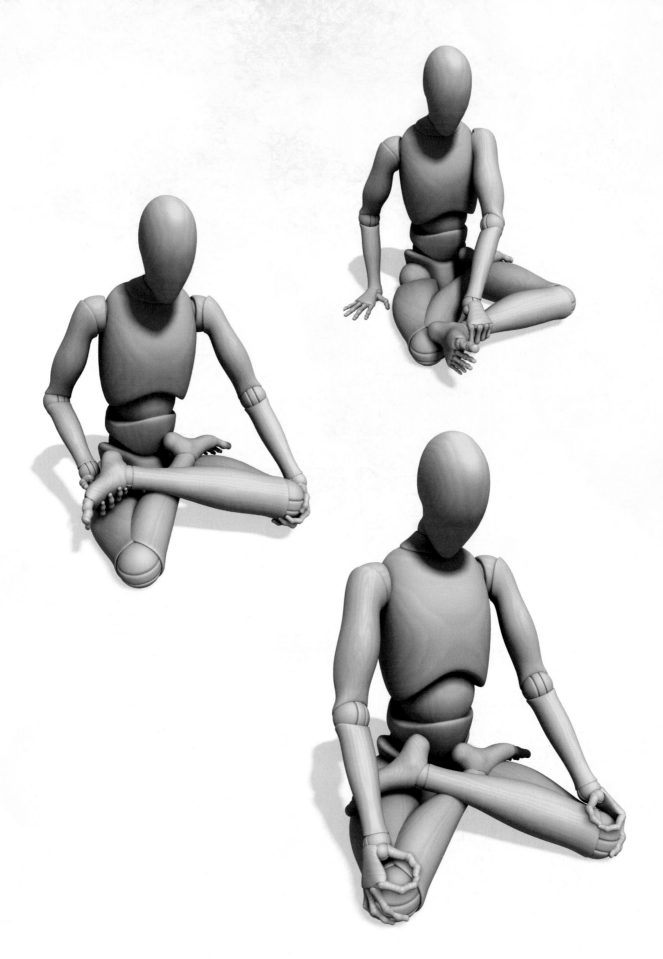

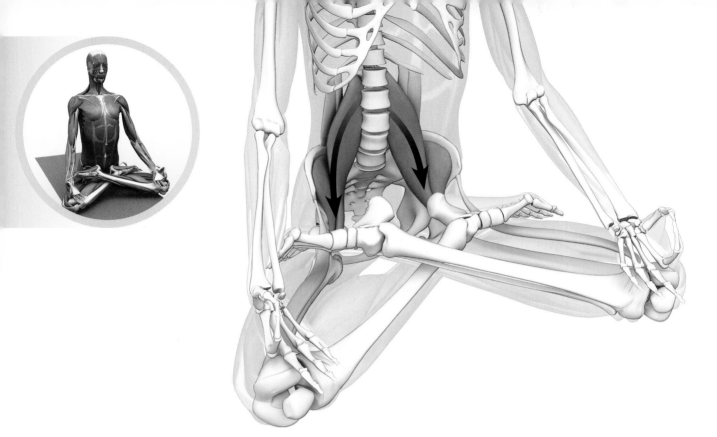

▲ **STEP 1** Flex the hips by engaging the psoas muscles. The cue for this is to press the palms onto the knees and gently attempt to lift up into the hands. This gives a feel for activating the psoas. Ideally, the knees rest in an abducted position so that contraction of the psoas is *closed chain* (the origin on the pelvis and lumbar spine moves, rather than the insertion on the femur). As a consequence, the pelvis tilts forward and the lumbar spine lifts and extends. The sartorius muscle, running from the anterior superior iliac spine to the inside of the knee, synergizes the tilt of the pelvis while aiding to abduct and externally rotate the hip.

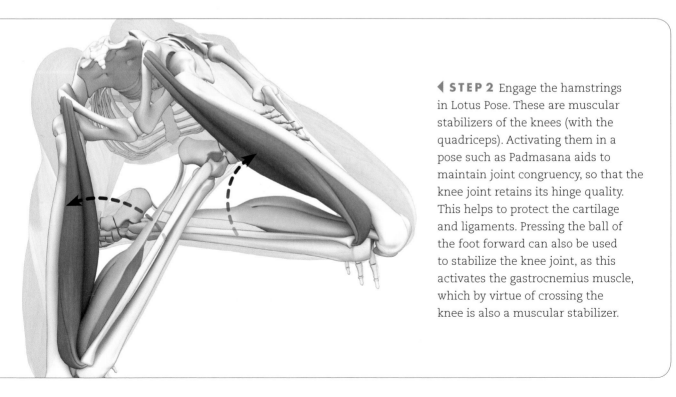

◀ **STEP 2** Engage the hamstrings in Lotus Pose. These are muscular stabilizers of the knees (with the quadriceps). Activating them in a pose such as Padmasana aids to maintain joint congruency, so that the knee joint retains its hinge quality. This helps to protect the cartilage and ligaments. Pressing the ball of the foot forward can also be used to stabilize the knee joint, as this activates the gastrocnemius muscle, which by virtue of crossing the knee is also a muscular stabilizer.

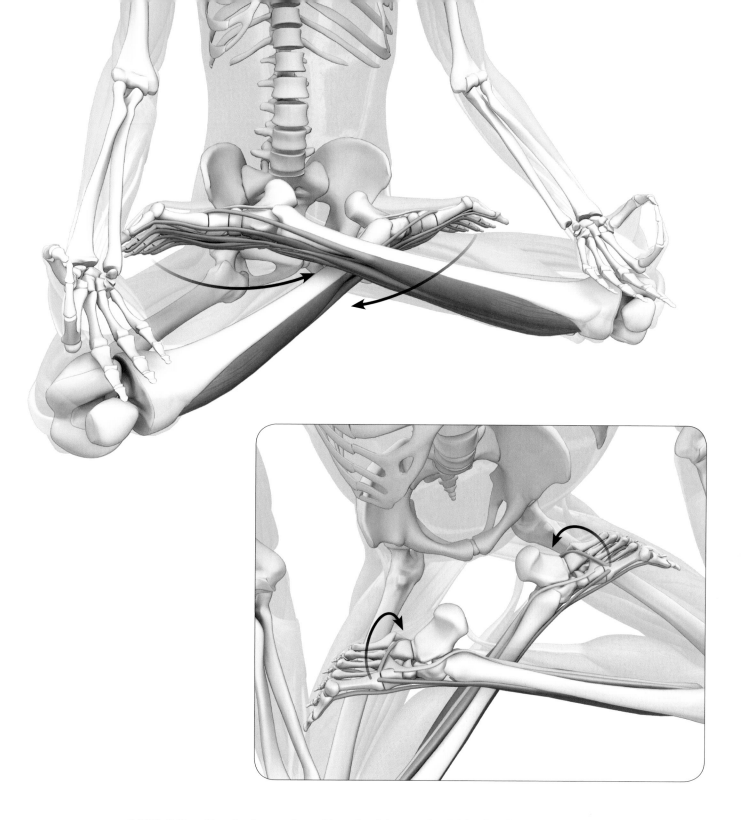

STEP 3 Dorsiflex the foot at the ankle to hook it onto the thigh. The tibialis anterior and toe extensors activate to create this action. Slightly evert the ankle as well by contracting the peroneus longus and brevis muscles on the lower side of the leg. This aids to protect the ligaments on the outside of the ankle from overstretching. Then balance eversion with a slight inversion force by activating the tibialis posterior. Note how these muscles combine to dynamize the longitudinal foot arch, as shown. Repeat on the other leg.

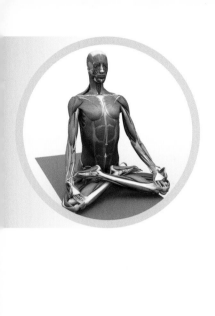

STEP 4 Tuck the tailbone under to engage the deep external hip rotators and the pubococcygeus muscle of the pelvic diaphragm. Activate the abductors at the sides of the hips—the gluteus medius and tensor fascia lata—to draw the thighs toward the floor.

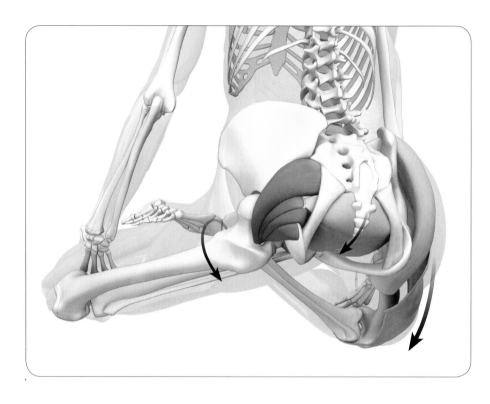

◀ **STEP 5** Externally rotate the shoulders by engaging the infraspinatus and teres minor muscles of the rotator cuff. The posterior deltoids (not shown) synergize this action. Press the hands into the knees and rotate the hands outward to activate these muscles (imagine the motion of washing a window).

Draw the shoulders away from the neck by contracting the lower third of the trapezius. Then adduct the scapulae toward the midline with the rhomboids. Hold the shoulders in this position to prepare for expanding the chest.

STEP 6 With the scapulae stabilized toward the midline of the back, attempt to roll the shoulders forward. The shoulders won't move, but the force of the action will engage the pectoralis minor and lift the ribcage. Expand the chest out to the sides by contracting the serratus anterior muscles on the sides of the ribcage. Visualize pushing the hands into a door frame to feel these muscles contract.

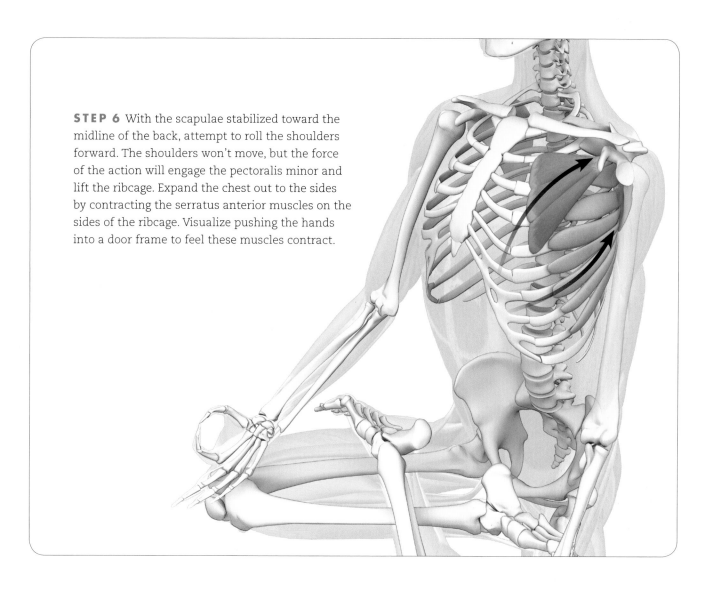

FORWARD
BENDS

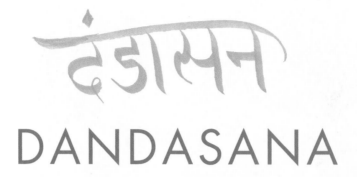

दंडासन

DANDASANA

STAFF POSE

DANDASANA CAN BE CONSIDERED A SEATED VARIANT OF TADASANA. IT SERVES as a barometer for the other seated poses, a place of return in which to assess the changes in the body and mind that are created by the preceding asana. The chest opens forward and up as in Tadasana. The hips flex to ninety degrees, and the lower back arches slightly. Initially, the tendency is to round the lower back and slump forward. This is generally due to some level of tightness in the muscles around the hips, including the hamstrings. To better understand why tight hamstrings would cause the lower back to round, look at the origin of the hamstrings from the ischial tuberosities of the pelvis. Tight hamstrings pull on these structures, causing the pelvis to tuck under (retrovert). This position of the pelvis then affects the lumbar spine, causing it to round. This is an example of coupled movement between the femur and pelvis and between the pelvis and vertebral column. Create length in the hamstrings in other poses, and then note how it becomes easier to align the vertebral column over the pelvis and sit up straight in Dandasana.

BASIC JOINT POSITIONS

- The hips flex.
- The knees extend.
- The ankles are neutral.
- The feet evert.
- The trunk extends.

- The shoulders adduct and externally rotate.
- The elbows extend.
- The forearms pronate.
- The wrists extend.

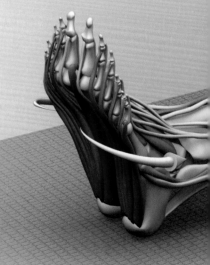

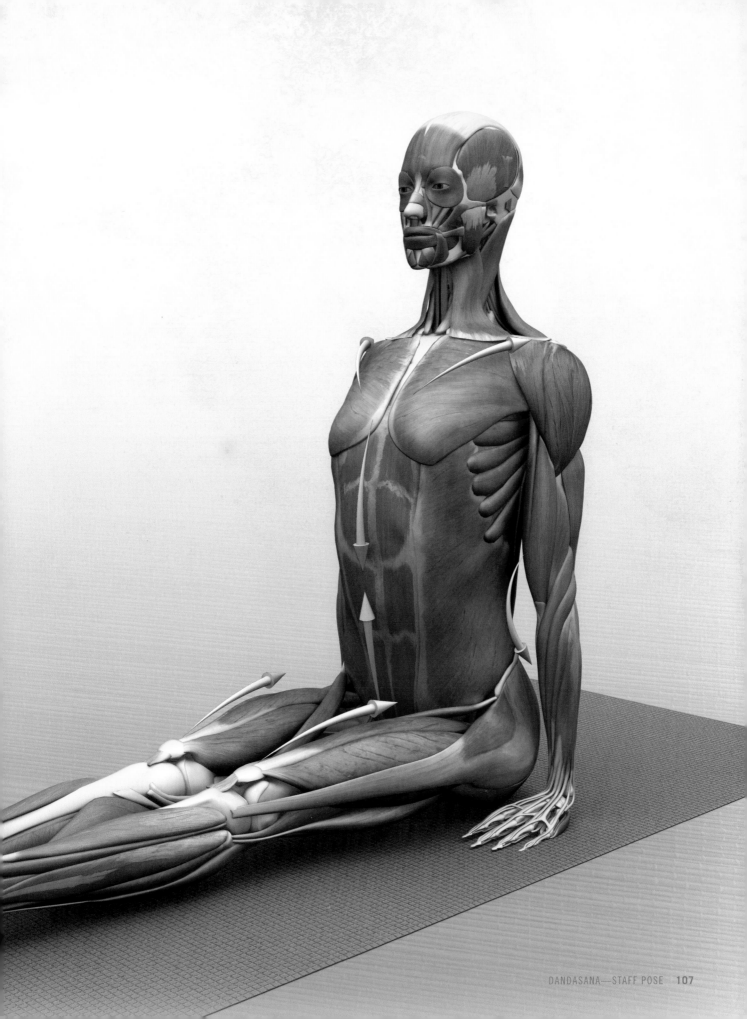

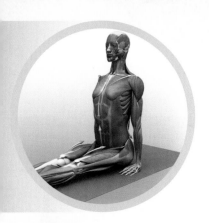

Dandasana Preparation

There can be a tendency to slump in Dandasana. You can address this by bending the knees to release the hamstrings. Notice how this frees you to extend the lower back. Engage the muscles surrounding the lumbar spine to maintain this position. Press the hands down and lift the chest. Then straighten the knees. If your back muscles feel tight, use forward bends such as Paschimottanasana to prepare for Dandasana.

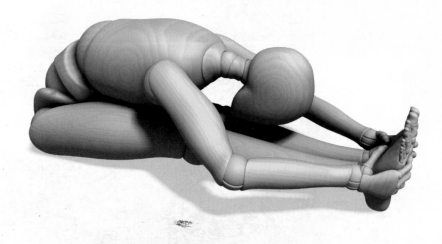

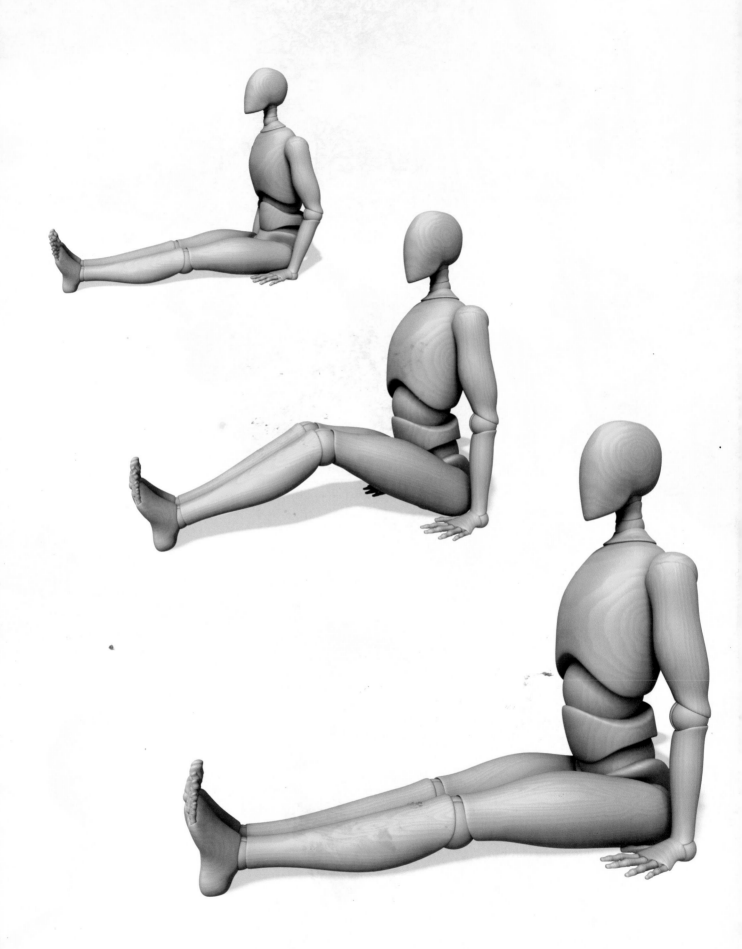

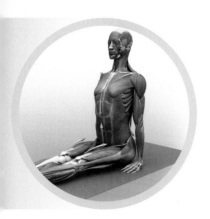

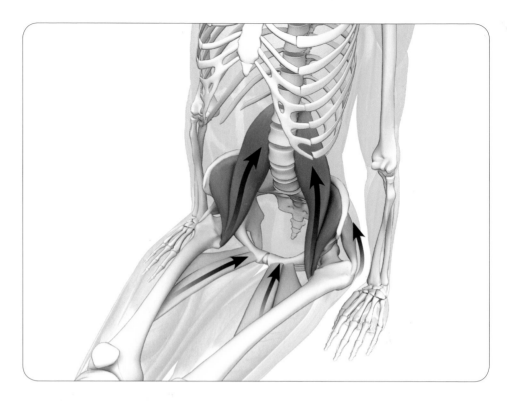

STEP 1 Flex the hips by engaging the psoas muscles. A cue for this action is to press the hands onto the thighs, squeeze the legs together, and attempt to lift them off the ground. This allows you to feel the psoas contracting. Two muscles wrap around and support the lumbar spine—the psoas major and the quadratus lumborum. The psoas major acts to draw the lumbar spine forward. This action takes place in concert with the quadratus lumborum due to a neurological connection between the two muscles, so that they are stimulated simultaneously to support the lumbar spine. The pelvis tilts forward as the lumbar spine extends and lifts. The anterior tilt of the pelvis combines with the flexion of the femurs, illustrating coupled movement between adjacent joints. The pectineus and adductors longus and brevis synergize flexing the femurs while drawing them together.

STEP 2 Straighten the knees by engaging the quadriceps. The sartorius and rectus femoris cross the hips, synergizing the quadriceps to extend the knees. Engage the tensor fascia lata, gluteus minimus, and anterior fibers of the gluteus medius to internally rotate the thighs. Adjust the rotation of the legs so that the kneecaps face directly upward and do not roll out to the side. A cue for engaging these muscles is to press the heels into the mat and attempt to drag them apart. Note how this action turns the thighs inward.

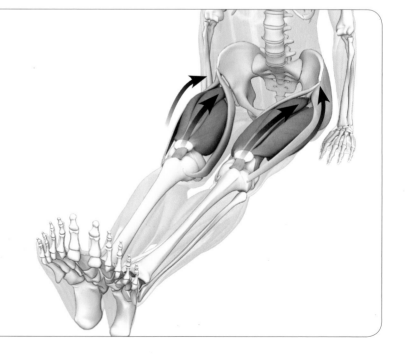

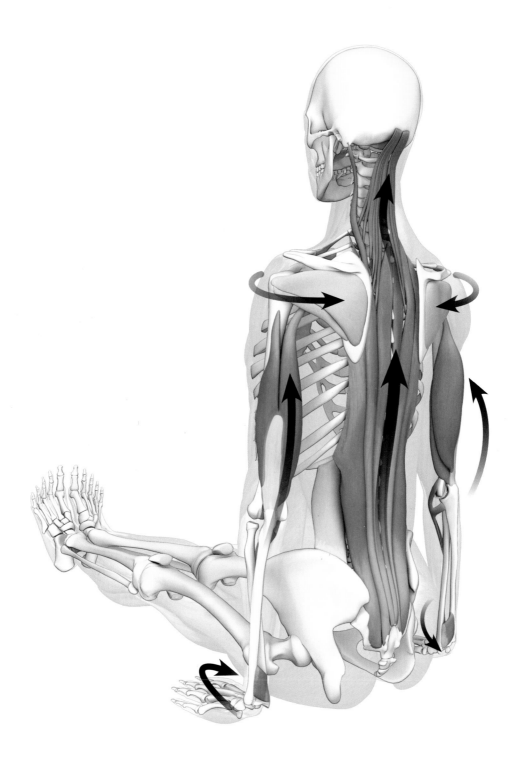

STEP 3 Several actions conspire to lift the back in Dandasana. The erector spinae and quadratus lumborum act directly on the vertebral column, extending it. Slightly arch the back to engage these muscles. Press the hands into the floor by contracting the triceps to extend the elbows. Then rotate the shoulders outward. This activates the infraspinatus and teres minor muscles of the rotator cuff. Press the mounds at the base of the index fingers into the floor to engage the pronators teres and quadratus of the forearms. The actions of the arms and shoulders will indirectly lift the spine and synergize the back muscles.

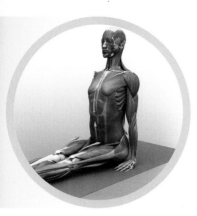

STEP 4 Draw the chest forward and up. Several muscles, including the latissimus dorsi, posterior deltoids, and rhomboids, work together to perform this action. The latissimus dorsi originates along the midline of the back, from the lumbopelvic area to the mid-thorax, and inserts on the upper humerus. We usually think of this muscle as drawing the humerus from a flexed to an extended position, as with a chin-up. This is known as open chain contraction of the muscle, wherein the insertion on the humerus moves but the origin remains relatively stationary. We can fix the hands on the mat so that the arms—the insertions of the latissimus dorsi—cannot move. Then, if we attempt to scrub the hands backwards on the mat, the latissimus dorsi contracts and moves its origin, lifting the back and expanding the chest. The posterior deltoids synergize this effect. Contract the rhomboids as well to draw the shoulder blades toward the midline. Stabilize them in place to prepare for the next step in the pose.

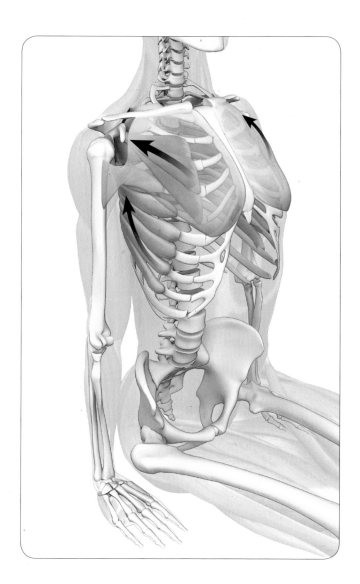

STEP 5 Contract the pectoralis minor to lift and open the ribcage. To engage this muscle, first fix the shoulder blades in place by activating the rhomboids (Step 4). Maintain the scapulae drawn back toward the midline, and then attempt to roll the shoulders forward. The pectoralis minor originates from the coracoid process of the scapula (the beak-like bone on the front of the shoulder blade). Since the rhomboids are preventing the scapulae from moving, the origin of the pectoralis minor remains stationary. The contraction of this muscle is transmitted to its insertion on the ribcage, lifting and expanding the chest. A similar process takes place with the pectoralis major. Finally, contract the serratus anterior to expand the chest out to the sides. As with the pectoralis minor, the origin of the serratus anterior is held in place by keeping the scapulae drawn back. Consequently, when we engage this muscle, the ribcage lifts and the chest expands.

STEP 6 Engage the péroneus longus and brevis muscles on the outsides of the lower legs to evert the soles of the feet. Draw the toes toward the head by activating the toe extensors. This begins to lift the arches. Engage the tibialis posterior to further lift the foot arch and stabilize the ankle. This muscle bridges the tibia and fibula, crosses the ankle, and inserts onto the inner surface of the midfoot. Visualize this muscle contracting to invert the feet and oppose the action of the peronei.

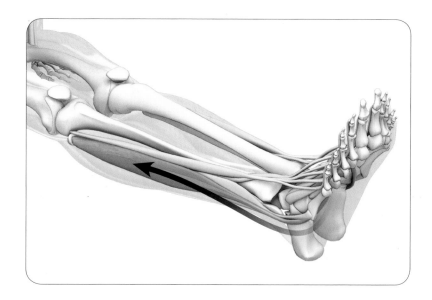

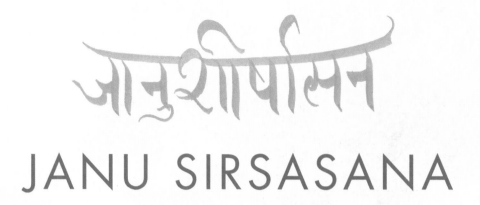

JANU SIRSASANA

HEAD-TO-KNEE POSE

THE MAIN STORY IN JANU SIRSASANA IS AN ASYMMETRICAL STRETCH OF THE posterior kinetic chain, including the muscles at the back of the straight leg and the back itself. Two subplots contribute to the main stretch. One is the action of the bent leg and the other is the action of the arms. In the bent leg, the femur flexes, abducts, and externally rotates, drawing that side of the pelvis away from the straight leg. Although the main focus is on the extended leg, periodically bring your attention to the flexed knee. Look at the muscles that produce the positions of the hip and knee on this side. Engage these muscles to make the pose more active. Grasp the foot with the hands to link the shoulder and pelvic girdles, transmitting a stretch from the back into the leg. Connect the action of the bent leg with the same-side arm. For example, as the bent knee draws back, flex the same-side elbow more. This creates two counterbalancing forces with simultaneous movements in different directions. We saw this concept in the warrior postures, with the back foot constrained as the front of the body lunges forward. Observe the effect of flexing the trunk while moving the bent knee back. Note that when the trunk flexes, the muscles and ligaments of the back pull on the pelvis, tilting it forward. Similarly, as the femur flexes, the pelvis tilts forward. In this way, both the trunk and hip work together to affect the hamstring muscles of the straight leg. Conversely, the hamstring muscles, which pull on the ischial tuberosities, affect the orientation of the pelvis. As these muscles gain length, the lumbar spine flexes less and the pelvis tilts forward more.

Note how the bent-leg side of the trunk is longer than the straight-leg side. To balance this, flex the elbow on the bent-leg side to lengthen the trunk on the straight-leg side.

BASIC JOINT POSITIONS

- The straight-leg hip flexes.
- The knee extends.
- The ankle plantar flexes.
- The foot everts.
- The bent-leg hip flexes, abducts, and externally rotates.

- The trunk flexes.
- The shoulders flex, abduct, and externally rotate.
- The elbows flex.
- The forearms pronate.
- The wrists extend.

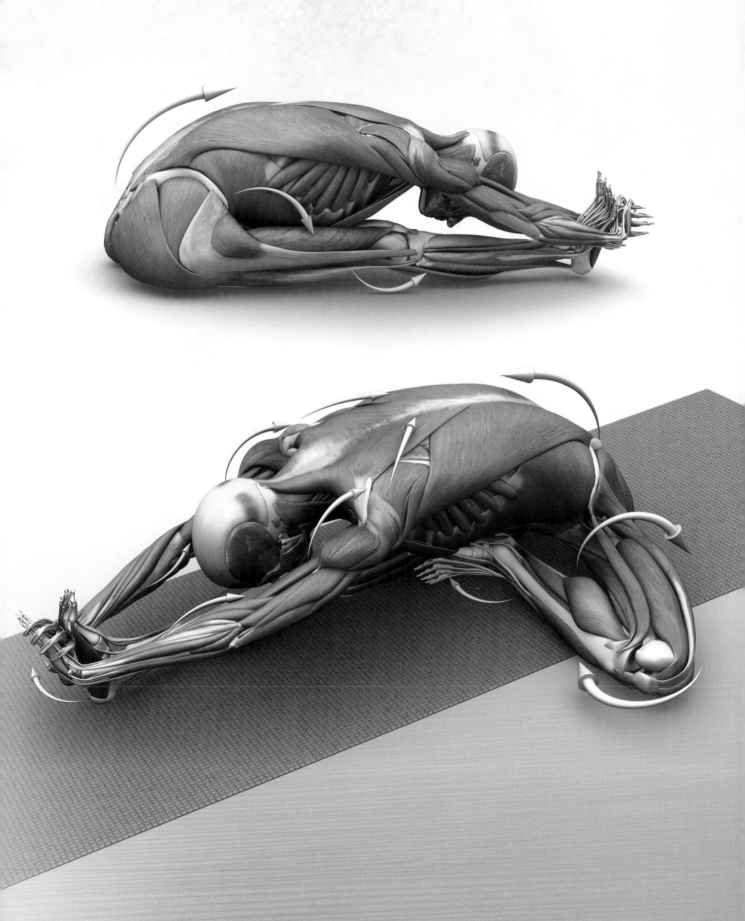

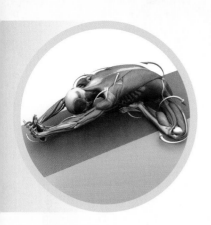

Janu Sirsasana Preparation

The posterior kinetic chain links the muscles, tendons, and ligaments at the back of the body. Tightness in one muscle affects the position of the joints in other muscles; for example, tightness in the lower back can make it difficult to straighten the knees, and tightness in the hamstrings can make it difficult to flex the trunk. Identify areas of inflexibility and modify the pose to accommodate these regions. Then use facilitated stretching to create length in the muscles that limit mobility.

Bend the knee and use a belt if necessary to link the hands to the foot. As the muscles lengthen (take as much time as needed), straighten the knee. Use your physiological reflexes to gain length in the muscles and mobility in the joints. Work within your limitations, and do not force progress. Use the cradle pose to stretch the tensor fascia lata and gluteal muscles to create length to externally rotate the femur.

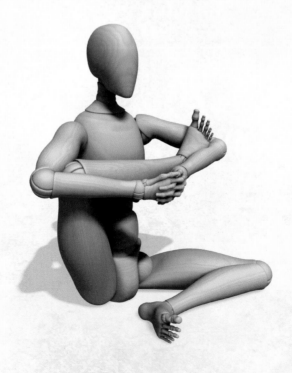

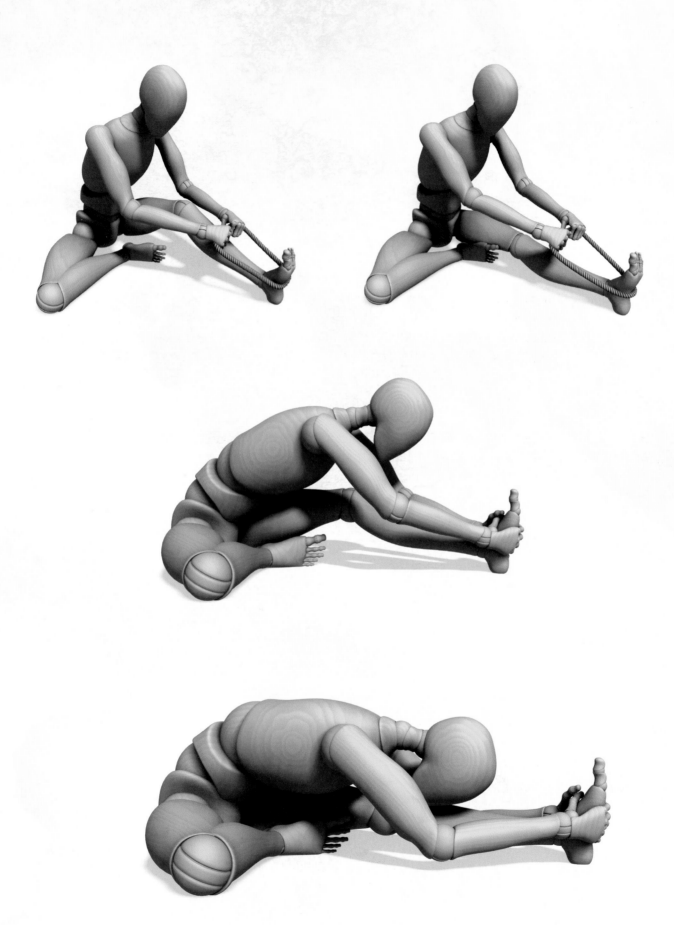

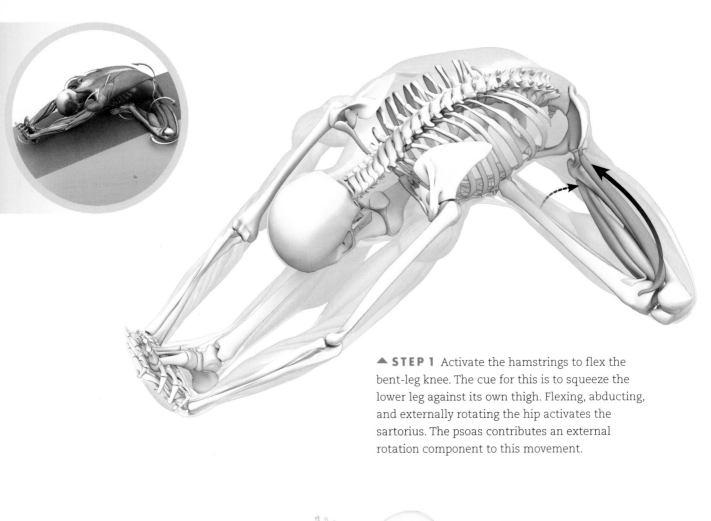

▲ **STEP 1** Activate the hamstrings to flex the
bent-leg knee. The cue for this is to squeeze the
lower leg against its own thigh. Flexing, abducting,
and externally rotating the hip activates the
sartorius. The psoas contributes an external
rotation component to this movement.

▶ **STEP 2** The gluteals and tensor fascia lata work together
in Janu Sirsasana. Squeeze the buttocks to engage the gluteus
maximus. This externally rotates and extends the hip, drawing
the bent knee back and down. Maintain joint congruency,
especially in the knee. With this in mind, maintain the knee
as a hinge and gain your rotation from the hip. Rotate the
thigh and lower leg as one unit, like a log. Use the gluteus
medius and tensor fascia lata to abduct the thigh out
to the side, drawing the knee back and down.

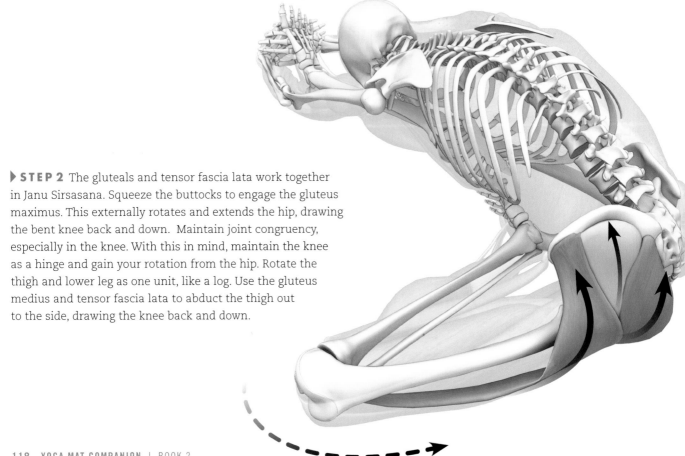

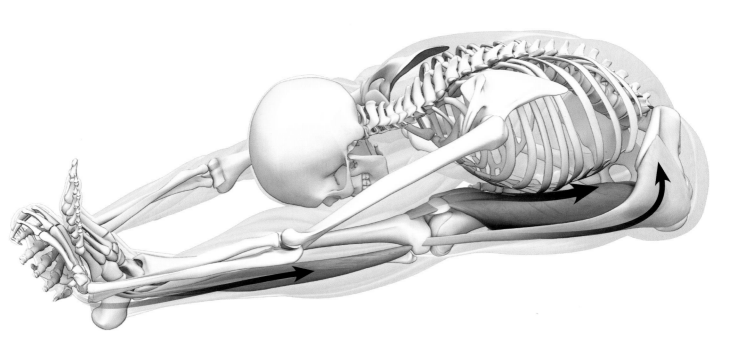

▲ **STEP 3** Contract the quadriceps to straighten the knee. The tensor fascia lata helps stabilize the outer side of the knee and aids to flex the hip. Notice how the hamstrings relax and feel different in the stretch when you actively engage the quadriceps, their antagonist. Engage the peroneus longus and brevis muscles on the side of the lower leg to turn the foot out and open the sole.

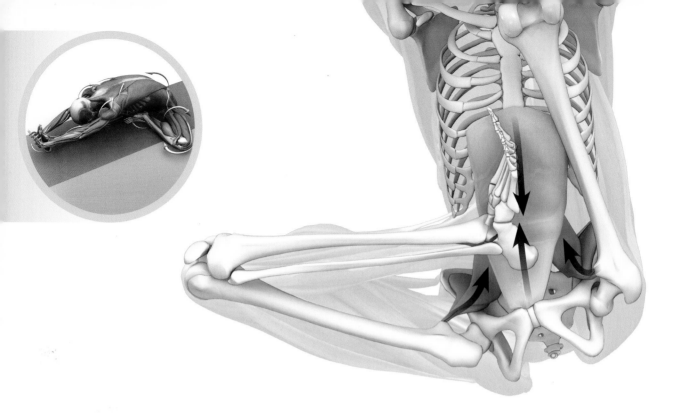

STEP 4 Squeeze the torso against the thigh to engage the psoas. Activate the abdominals to flex and turn the bent-leg side of the trunk. Experience how this action changes the feeling of the stretch in the lower back muscles, including the quadratus lumborum. This is a result of reciprocal inhibition. Note that when the femur flexes, the pelvis tilts forward—an example of coupled movement within the hip. Compare this with how flexing, abducting, and externally rotating the bent-leg hip tilts that side of the pelvis back and down. Tilting the pelvis in opposite directions creates a "wringing" effect across the sacroiliac ligaments and produces a stabilizing bandha in this region.

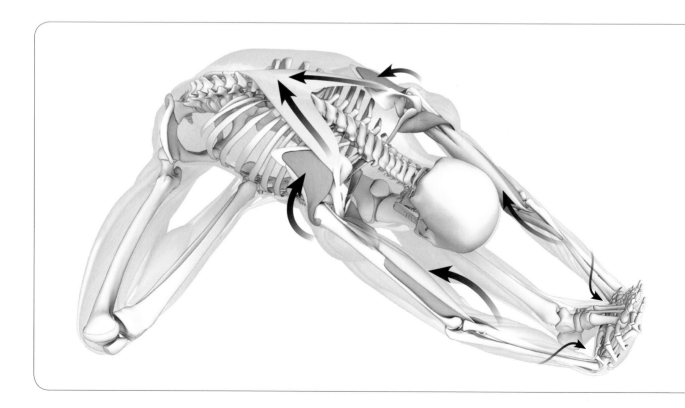

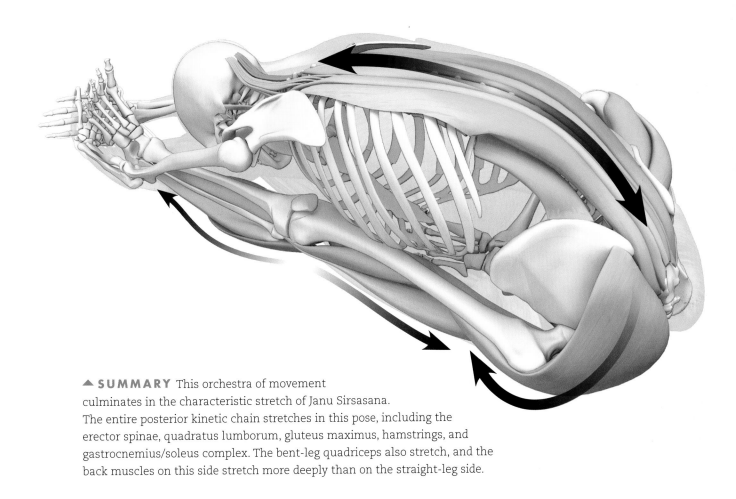

SUMMARY This orchestra of movement culminates in the characteristic stretch of Janu Sirsasana. The entire posterior kinetic chain stretches in this pose, including the erector spinae, quadratus lumborum, gluteus maximus, hamstrings, and gastrocnemius/soleus complex. The bent-leg quadriceps also stretch, and the back muscles on this side stretch more deeply than on the straight-leg side.

◀ **STEP 5** Connecting the upper and lower extremities allows you to use the force generated by the arms to stretch the muscles of the back and lower leg. Contract the biceps and brachialis to bend the elbows and draw the trunk further over the leg. Flex the elbow more strongly on the bent-leg side to draw that side of the body more toward the extended leg, stretching the side of the body. If you are grasping the foot as shown, then pronate the forearms by pressing the mounds at the base of the index fingers forward. Engage the infraspinatus and teres minor muscles to rotate the shoulders outward. Fix the hands on the feet and attempt to raise the arms up. This contracts the anterior deltoids and draws the trunk deeper. Finally, draw the shoulders away from the ears by engaging the lower portions of the trapezius.

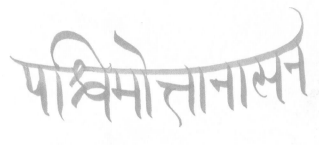

PASCHIMOTTANASANA

INTENSE STRETCH TO THE WEST POSE

THE MAIN STORY IN PASCHIMOTTANASANA IS A SYMMETRICAL STRETCH OF THE BACK of the body, especially the hamstrings. Look at how this pose is different from an asymmetrical pose, such as Janu Sirsasana.

Everything starts with the pelvis. For example, in Janu Sirsasana, the pelvis tilts and angles and the hips are relatively diagonal to each other. Moving outward from the pelvis, the bent-leg hip is directed back and away from the body and is externally rotated. This angling of the pelvis affects the curvature of the spine, which in turn affects the position of the shoulders, and so on.

In Paschimottanasana, on the other hand, the pelvis is in a neutral position and the hip joints are relatively in line with each other. Paschimottanasana folds the body forward, flexing both the trunk and the hips. The knees extend, and the hands grasp the feet to link the upper and lower appendicular skeletons. The shoulder and pelvic girdles are connected by the vertebral column; thus actions in the shoulders and hips conspire to affect the spine and back, which in turn influence the position of the pelvis. This is an example of triangulation, wherein two points—here the shoulder and pelvic girdles—affect and are influenced by another point—the spinal column. Flexing the trunk causes the muscles, tendons, and ligaments of the back to pull upward on the pelvis, tilting it forward. This action draws the origins of the hamstrings on the ischial tuberosities up and back, stretching these muscles.

BASIC JOINT POSITIONS

- The hips flex.
- The knees extend.
- The ankles plantar flex.
- The feet evert.
- The trunk flexes.

- The shoulders flex, abduct, and externally rotate.
- The elbows flex.
- The forearms pronate.
- The wrists extend.

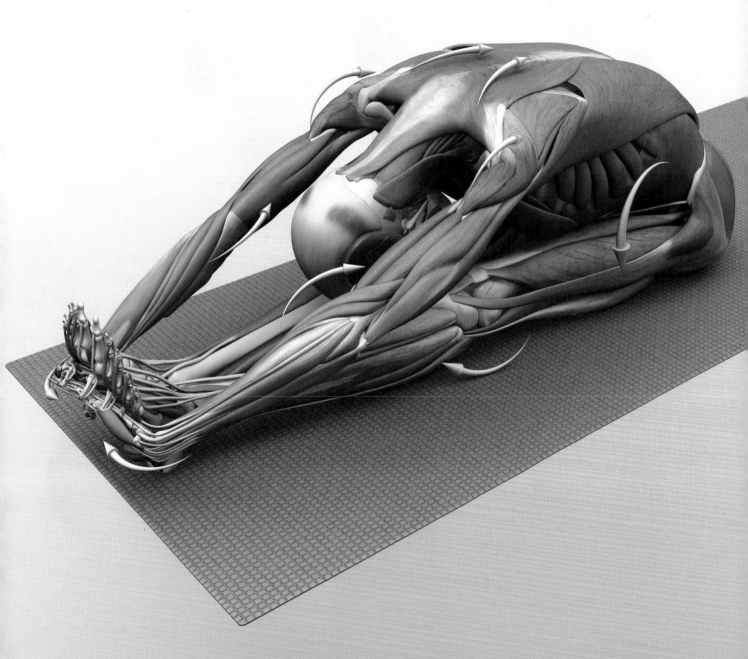

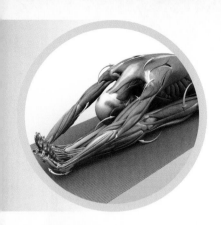

Paschimottanasana Preparation

If your hamstring or back muscles are tight, feel free to use a belt. Begin with the knees bent. Then activate the quadriceps to straighten the knees, and flex the elbows to draw the torso over the thighs. Squeeze the thighs together by engaging the adductor muscles, and turn the sides of the feet slightly outward to open the soles. As you gain flexibility, reach forward to grasp the lower legs or feet, and then bend the elbows more to draw the upper body deeper into the pose. Use a standing forward bend such as Uttanasana to prepare the hamstrings and back muscles for the stretch from a different orientation. This takes advantage of the direction of gravity, so that the weight of the torso pulls on the posterior kinetic chain and further anteverts the pelvis to stretch the hamstrings.

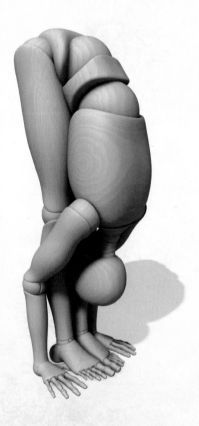

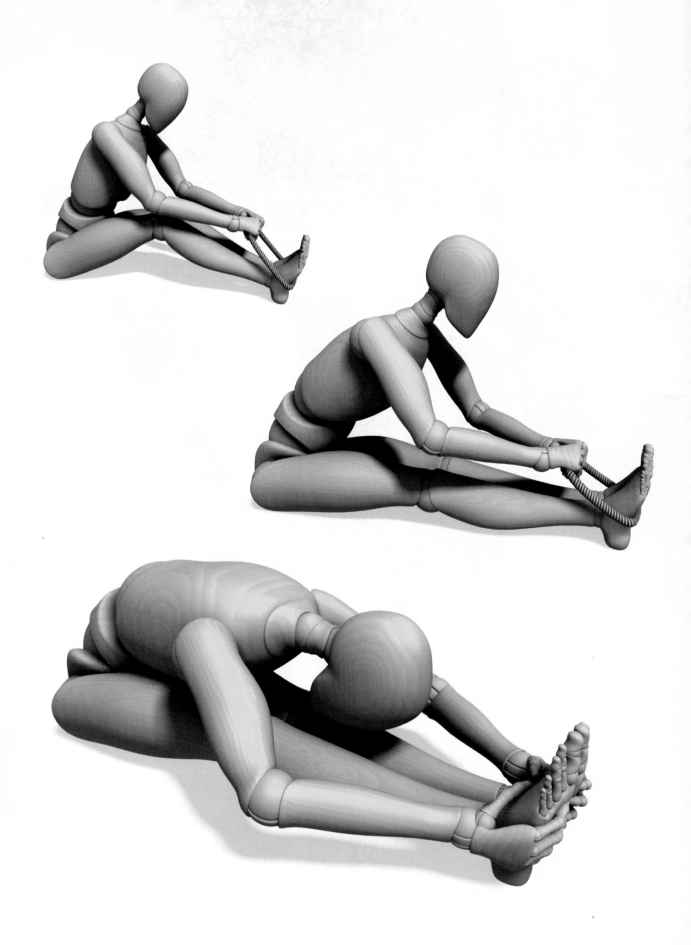

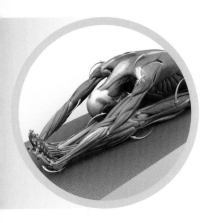

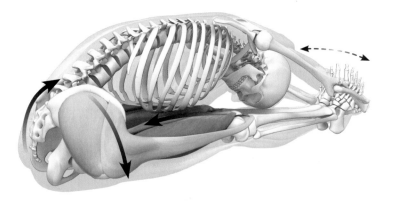

STEP 1 Contract the quadriceps to straighten the knees, creating reciprocal inhibition of the hamstrings. The rectus femoris and tensor fascia lata cross the hip joint and contribute to flexing the femurs while synergizing the action of straightening the knees. As the femurs flex, the pelvis anteverts, or tilts forward. Press the sides of the feet into the hands to engage the gluteus medius and tensor fascia lata. The force of this contraction will aid to release the sacroiliac joint, allowing the spine to flex deeper into the pose. This is an example of nutation of the sacrum. You can also visualize the gluteus minimus synergizing hip flexion.

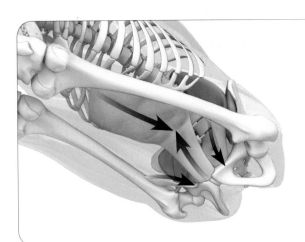

◄ STEP 2 Contract the abdominals to flex the trunk. This creates reciprocal inhibition of the back muscles, allowing them to relax into the stretch. The psoas flexes the femurs and draws the trunk onto the thighs. This muscle curves over the front of the pelvis and tilts it forward (anteversion). The rectus abdominis attaches on the pubic symphysis and tilts the pelvis back (retroversion); accordingly, the rectus abdominis and psoas work together to stabilize the pelvis by virtue of their opposing actions.

▶ STEP 3 Activate the biceps and brachialis muscles to bend the elbows and draw the trunk further over the thighs. If your hands reach around the feet as shown, then contract the pronators teres and quadratus to evert the palms and turn them outward. Alternatively, if your palms face the trunk as you grasp the sides of the feet, engage the supinator muscles of the forearms to attempt to turn the palms upward. Maintain the hands fixed on the feet and try to lift the arms straight up. Notice how this activates the anterior deltoids and draws the torso deeper into the pose. Hold the elbows up so that the arm bones are parallel to the floor, and rotate the shoulders externally, using the infraspinatus and teres minor muscles. Draw the shoulders away from the ears with the lower trapezius. These actions lengthen the entire posterior kinetic chain at the back of the body.

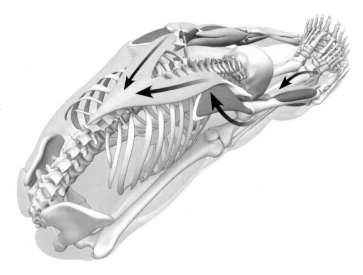

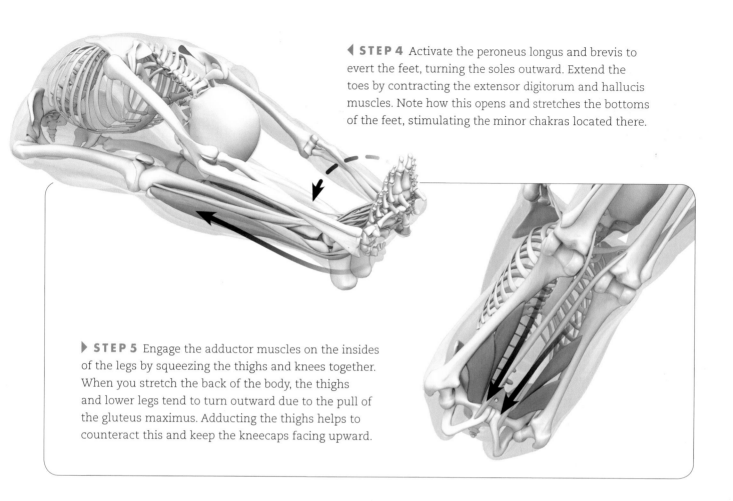

◀ **STEP 4** Activate the peroneus longus and brevis to evert the feet, turning the soles outward. Extend the toes by contracting the extensor digitorum and hallucis muscles. Note how this opens and stretches the bottoms of the feet, stimulating the minor chakras located there.

▶ **STEP 5** Engage the adductor muscles on the insides of the legs by squeezing the thighs and knees together. When you stretch the back of the body, the thighs and lower legs tend to turn outward due to the pull of the gluteus maximus. Adducting the thighs helps to counteract this and keep the kneecaps facing upward.

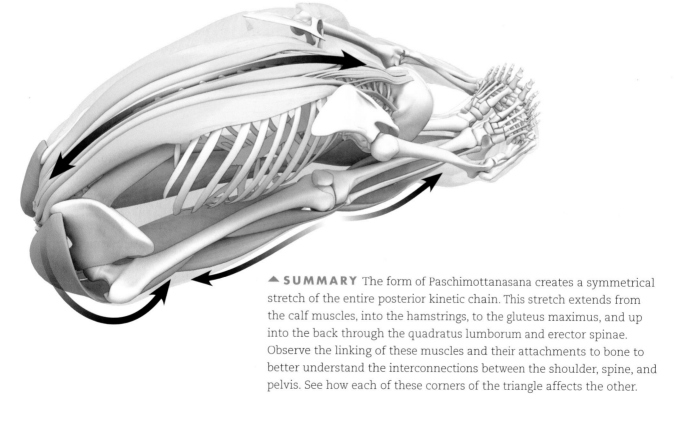

▲ **SUMMARY** The form of Paschimottanasana creates a symmetrical stretch of the entire posterior kinetic chain. This stretch extends from the calf muscles, into the hamstrings, to the gluteus maximus, and up into the back through the quadratus lumborum and erector spinae. Observe the linking of these muscles and their attachments to bone to better understand the interconnections between the shoulder, spine, and pelvis. See how each of these corners of the triangle affects the other.

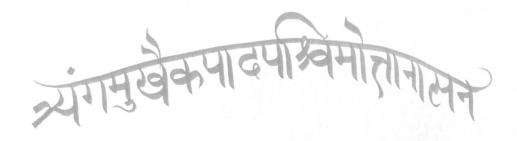

TRIANG MUKHAIKAPADA PASCHIMOTTANASANA

THREE LIMBS FACE ONE FOOT POSE

TRIANG MUKHAIKAPADA PASCHIMOTTANASANA CAN FEEL AWKWARD AND OFF balance. One knee is flexing alongside the body and the other leg extends forward, so that tipping to the side of the straight leg is nearly inevitable. How did the ancients come up with this pose?!

The main story here is a stretch of the back of the body, including the straight leg. However, there is a complex build-up to this main plot. In Triang Mukhaikapada Paschimottanasana, obtaining evenness in the pelvis precedes stretching the back side of the body. In any event, maintaining balance can be a struggle. This often leads to using a prop, such as a block or blanket, under the straight-leg buttocks. Props, like teachers, are bridges to working on your own. For example, place support under the straight-leg buttocks to push the body weight toward the bent-leg side, shifting the center of gravity. Then analyze how to create the same force of the prop using biomechanics and muscles alone. Begin by engaging the hip and knee flexors of the bent leg to draw the torso toward that leg. Then contract the abductors of the straight leg to synergize this action and push the body toward the midline. The cue for engaging these muscles is to fix the heel on the mat and attempt to "scrub" it to the side. The heel cannot move, so the force of the scrub shifts the body back toward the midline, preventing you from falling over. Once you attain balance in the pose, squeeze the knees together and bend forward.

BASIC JOINT POSITIONS

- The hips flex.
- The straight-leg knee extends.
- The ankle plantar flexes.
- The foot everts.
- The bent-leg knee flexes.
- The ankle plantar flexes.

- The trunk flexes.
- The shoulders flex, abduct, and externally rotate.
- The elbows flex.
- The forearms supinate.
- The wrists flex.

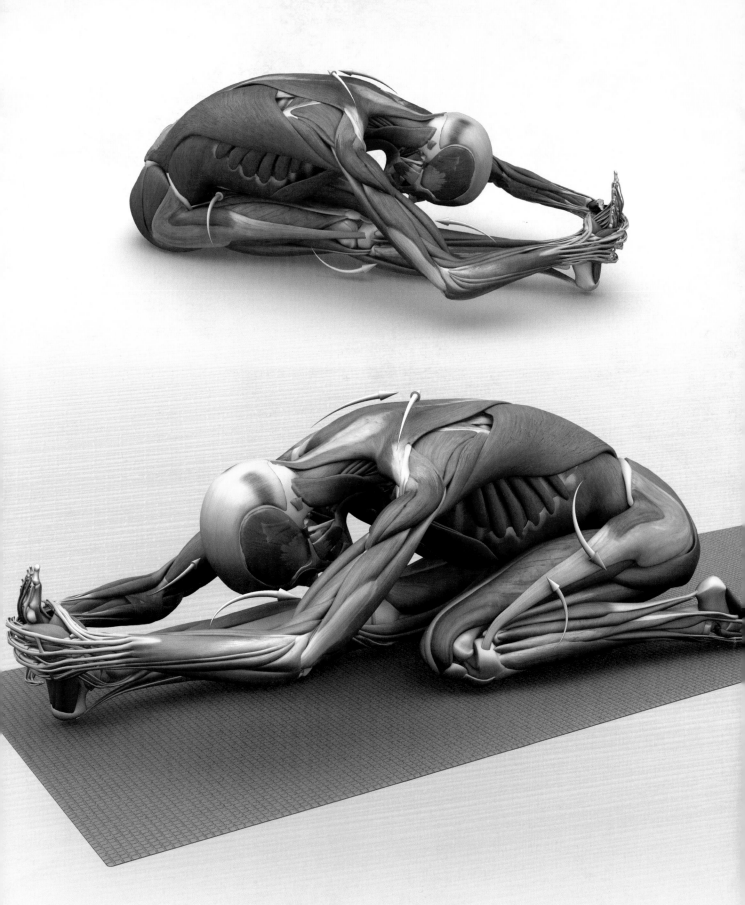

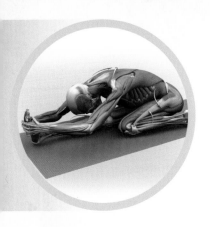

Triang Mukhaikapada
Paschimottanasana Preparation

Link the hands to the foot with a belt and bend the knee as shown. Use caution with the knee that is fully flexing. Sit on a block or a blanket to take some of the bend out of the joint if necessary. If you have pain in the knee, don't practice this pose. Activate the quadriceps to straighten the leg, and draw the body forward. As you gain flexibility, toss the belt aside and grasp the foot. Then straighten the knee to draw the trunk forward. Brace yourself to ease out of the pose: bend the straight leg and allow yourself to shift to the side while unfolding the bent knee.

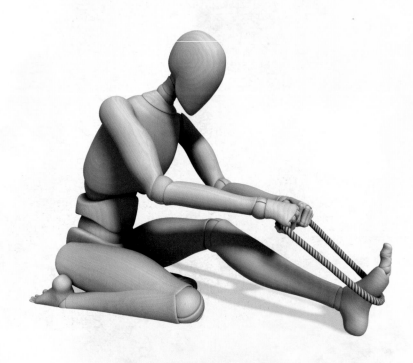

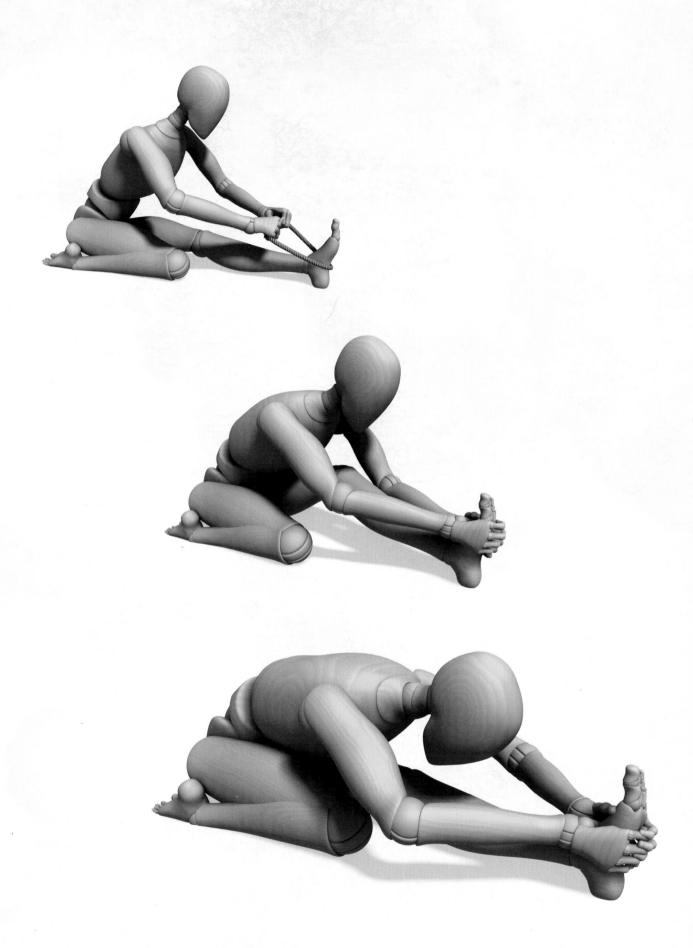

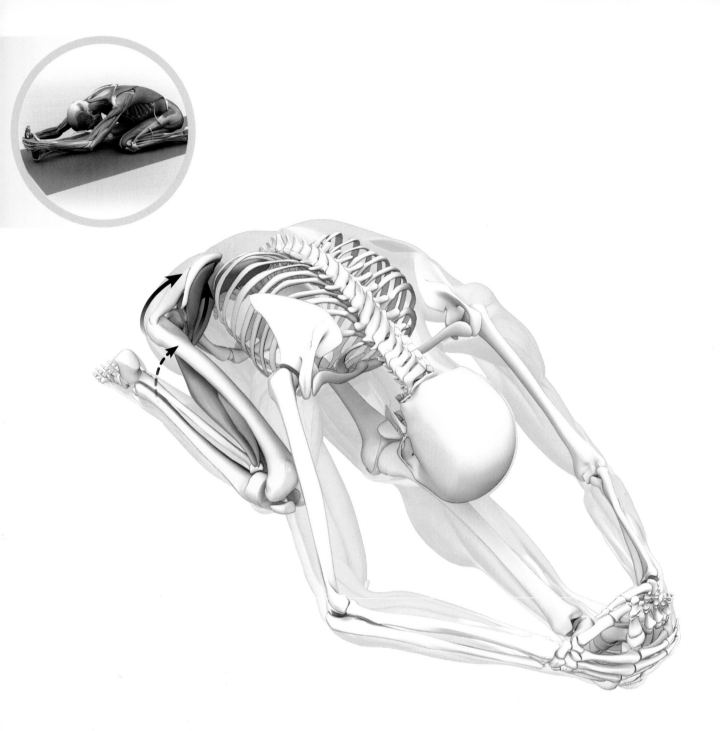

STEP 1 Flex the knee by contracting the hamstrings. The cue for this is to squeeze the lower leg into the upper one. Engaging these muscles also aids to protect the knee because the hamstrings are muscular stabilizers of that joint and draw the cartilage surfaces into congruency. Activate the psoas and gluteus minimus to flex the hip. A useful cue for engaging these muscles is to put the palm of the hand on the knee and press down while you attempt to raise it. You will feel the psoas contract. This closed chain contraction moves the origin of the psoas and tilts the pelvis forward. Notice how engaging these muscles draws the body toward the bent-leg side and grounds the pelvis. When the pelvis tilts forward, the ischial tuberosities (the origins of the hamstrings) move backward. This action augments the stretch of these muscles on the straight-leg side.

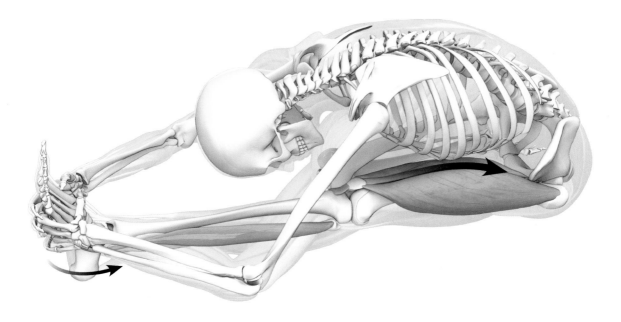

▲ **STEP 2** Activate the quadriceps of the straight leg to extend the knee. Evert the foot by engaging the peroneus longus and brevis along the side of the lower leg. The rectus femoris of the quadriceps crosses the hip and aids to flex it. Contracting the quadriceps also aids to release the hamstrings due to reciprocal inhibition.

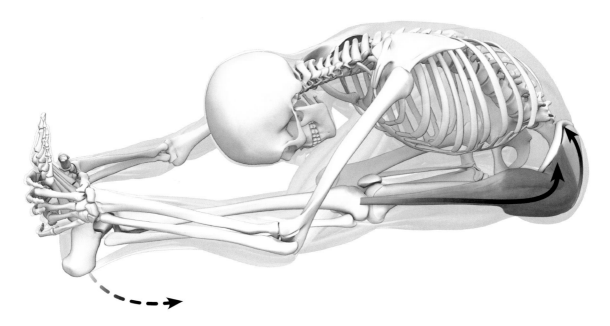

▲ **STEP 3** Push the body toward the bent knee by pressing the heel of the straight leg into the floor and attempting to drag it to the side. This cue activates the abductor muscles of the leg, including the gluteus medius and tensor fascia lata. The internal rotation component of the abductors counters the tendency of this foot to roll out to the side, bringing the kneecap to a neutral position, facing upward.

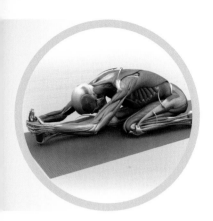

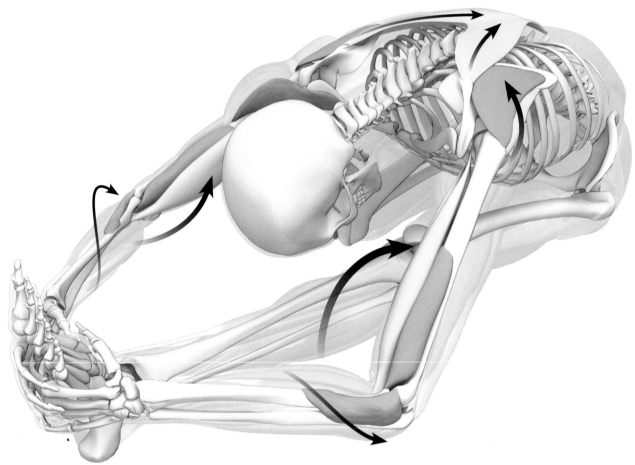

STEP 4 Contract the supinator muscles of the forearms to turn the palms and lock the grip. Bend the elbows by activating the biceps and brachialis muscles. Note that the biceps also aid to turn the palms. Grasp the feet and attempt to lift the hands straight up by engaging the anterior deltoids. Because the hands do not move, this action draws the torso deeper into the pose. Externally rotate the humeri while bringing the arm bones parallel to the floor. Draw the shoulders away from the neck with the lower third of the trapezius. All of these actions indirectly flex the trunk further into the stretch.

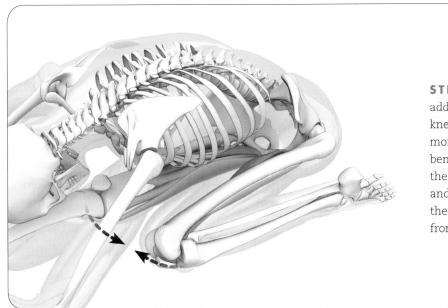

STEP 5 Engage the adductors to draw the knees together. Contract more forcefully on the bent-leg side to synergize the actions of the psoas and hamstrings in shifting the center of gravity away from the straight leg.

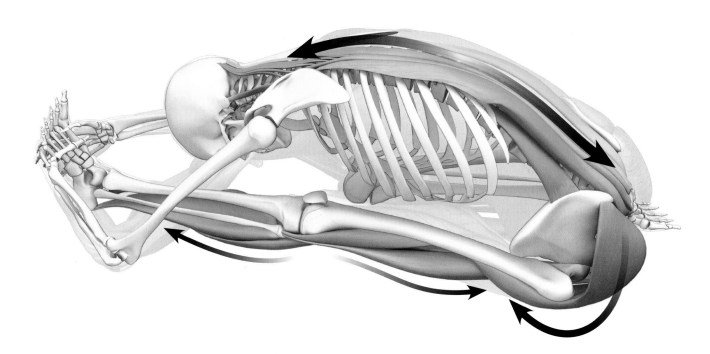

SUMMARY As with other forward-bending poses, Triang Mukhaikapada Paschimottanasana stretches the back of the body. It is an asymmetrical pose, with the back muscles on the bent-leg side stretching more deeply. The gluteus maximus, hamstrings, and gastrocnemius on the straight-leg side stretch in a manner similar to Janu Sirsasana. The bent-leg quadriceps also lengthen, except the rectus femoris. This muscle crosses the hip and is released in this pose.

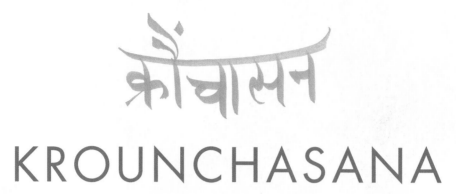

KROUNCHASANA

HERON POSE

KROUNCHASANA TAKES THE STORY OF TRIANG MUKHAIKAPADA PASCHIMOTTANASANA to another level. The most obvious new element is the lift of the straight leg into the air. This action provides several opportunities to apply our various techniques. As the hip of the straight leg flexes and the knee extends, the muscles at the back of the leg (those that flex the knee and extend the hip) stretch and draw the pelvis down and back into retroversion, rounding the back. Conversely, factors that tilt the pelvis forward—even just a little bit— draw the sitting bones back. This tweaks the pose because the ischial tuberosities are the origins of the same muscles that are lengthening, and moving these bones augments the stretch. To experience this, hold the foot of the straight leg with one hand and press down with the other hand onto the bent knee. Then attempt to lift that knee up against the hand (while resisting). This activates the hip flexors on this side of the pelvis and tilts it forward. Tilting the pelvis forward rotates the ischial tuberosities back slightly, pulling on the ham-string muscles at their origins and creating a unique type of stretch. You may need to try this more than once to get it.

There are several subplots to the pose as well. The arms draw the foot toward the body, and the abdominals flex the trunk forward. The breath in the background is the soundtrack.

BASIC JOINT POSITIONS

- The straight-leg hip flexes.
- The knee extends.
- The ankle plantar flexes.
- The foot everts.
- The bent-leg hip flexes.
- The ankle plantar flexes.

- The trunk flexes.
- The shoulders flex, abduct, and externally rotate.
- The elbows flex.
- The forearms supinate.
- The wrists flex.

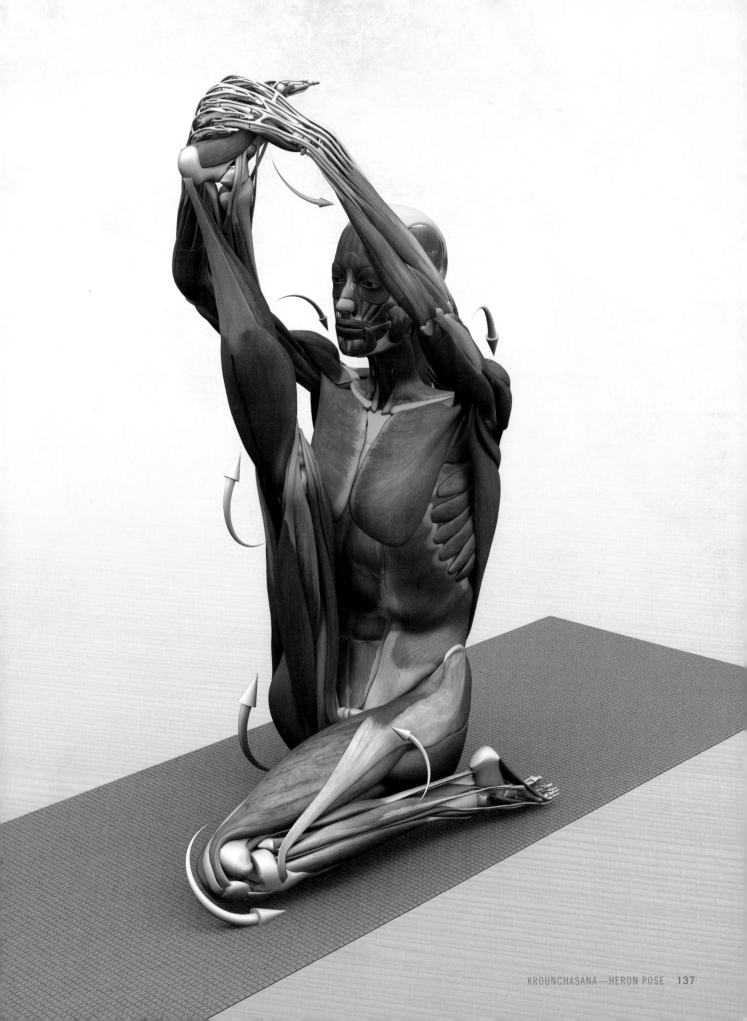

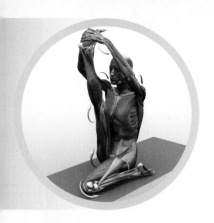

Krounchasana Preparation

Catch the foot with a belt, keeping the knee slightly flexed. If you have pain in the knee that is on the floor, you may try sitting on a blanket or block to take some of the flexion out of the joint. If the pain persists, then come out of the pose.

Get a feeling for raising the foot by lifting the arms and bending the elbows. Feel how this stretches the back of the leg. Draw the trunk toward the thigh, and attempt to hold it there while you activate the quadriceps to straighten the knee.

As you gain flexibility, you can reach forward and grasp the foot with your hands instead of a belt. Draw the thigh toward the trunk by bending the elbows. Feel how this stretches the back of the leg. Then activate the quadriceps to straighten the knee. This stimulates the reflex arc of reciprocal inhibition of the hamstrings, allowing them to relax into the stretch. Using only the leverage of the arms to straighten the leg (without contracting the quadriceps) stretches the hamstrings indirectly; it does not, however, stimulate reciprocal inhibition. This is why you have to activate the quadriceps, which are the antagonists to the hamstrings (the muscles being stretched).

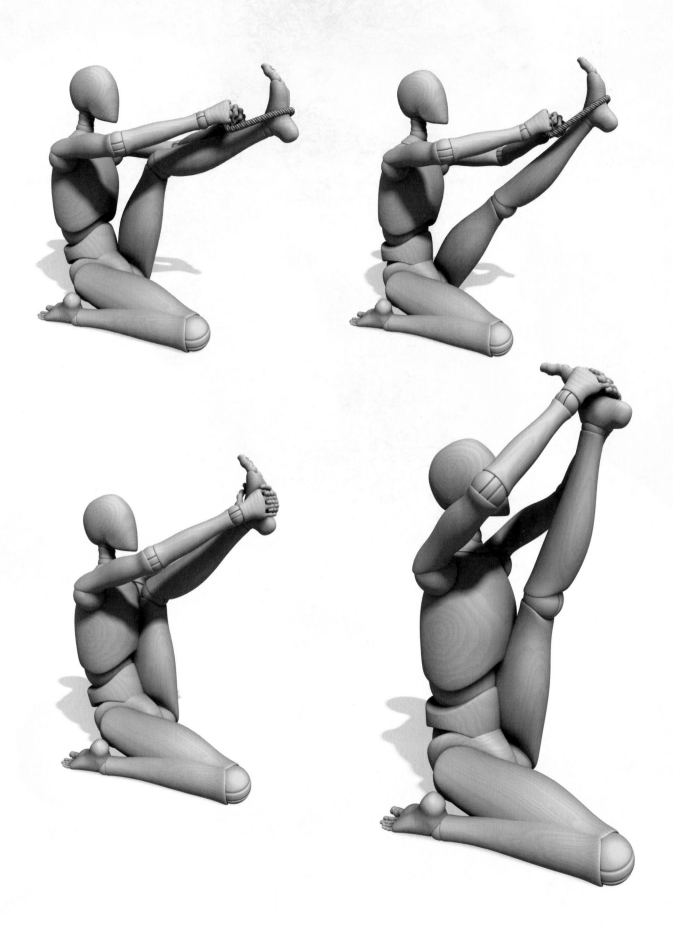

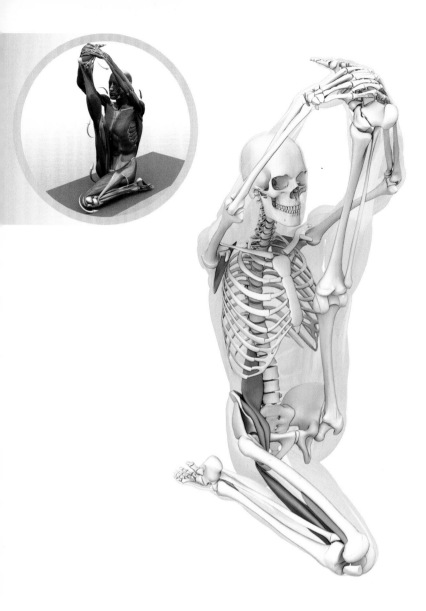

◀ **STEP 1** Contract the hamstrings to bend the knee. Squeeze the lower leg against the thigh as in Triang Mukhaikapada Paschimottanasana. Engaging the hamstrings helps to maintain congruency of the knee joint as a hinge. Press one hand onto the knee and attempt to lift it while resisting. This activates the psoas and its synergists of knee flexion in a closed chain fashion and anteverts the pelvis. Tilting the pelvis forward lengthens the hamstrings on the straight-leg side by rotating the ischial tuberosity up and back.

▶ **STEP 2** Use the psoas to draw the femur into the trunk. Note that when the hip is fully flexed, as in this pose, the psoas cannot produce much additional flexion force, as it is already fully contracted. Activate the rectus abdominis to flex the trunk. Remember the effect this has on nutation at the sacroiliac joint: it draws the pubic symphysis upward as the sacrum tilts forward (with flexion of the lumbar spine).

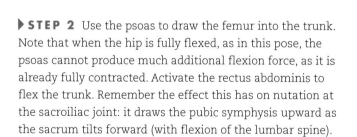

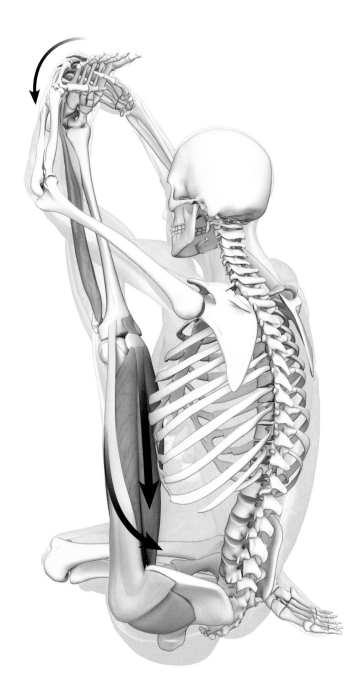

STEP 3 Engage the quadriceps to straighten the knee. This reciprocally inhibits the hamstrings from contracting in response to the stretch—a biomechanical and physiological yin/yang in yoga. This pose also stretches the gluteus maximus of the straight leg. Remember that the gluteus maximus extends and externally rotates the hip and femur. Stretching a muscle pulls on its attachments and can passively produce the same movements as when the muscle contracts. Thus flexing the hip stretches and pulls on the gluteus maximus, causing the thigh to roll out

in Krounchasana. Counteract this by engaging the gluteus medius and tensor fascia lata, two muscles that internally rotate the thigh. The cue for activating these muscles is to attempt to abduct the straight leg away from the midline while resisting with the hand. Abduction is another action of the gluteus medius and tensor fascia lata. You can use this cue to elicit the internal rotation action of these muscles and counteract the outward roll of the thigh produced by the stretching gluteus maximus. This illustrates the concept of dual muscle actions.

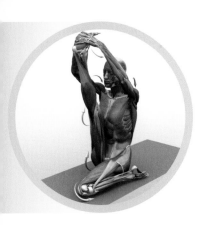

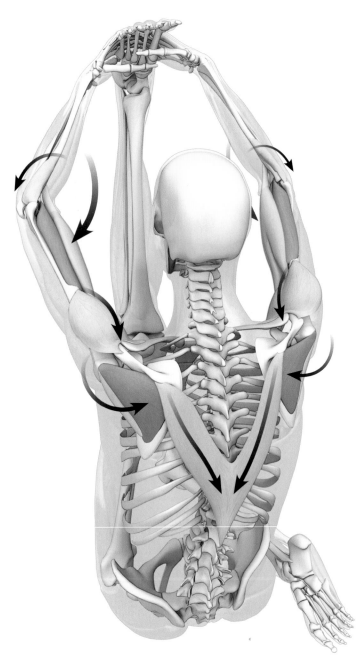

STEP 4 Grasp the foot to connect the upper and lower appendicular skeletons (the arms and the leg). Attempt to rotate the palms upward to lock the grip of the hands. This activates the supinator muscles. Contracting the biceps also supinates the forearms while bending the elbows (in synergy with the brachialis). Flex the wrists and firmly grasp the foot; then attempt to lift the arms upward, engaging the anterior deltoids. Note how this draws the leg toward the trunk and the trunk toward the leg. Create a "wringing" helical effect down the arms by externally rotating the shoulders with the infraspinatus and teres minor muscles. Activate the lower trapezius to draw the shoulders away from the ears and lift the chest.

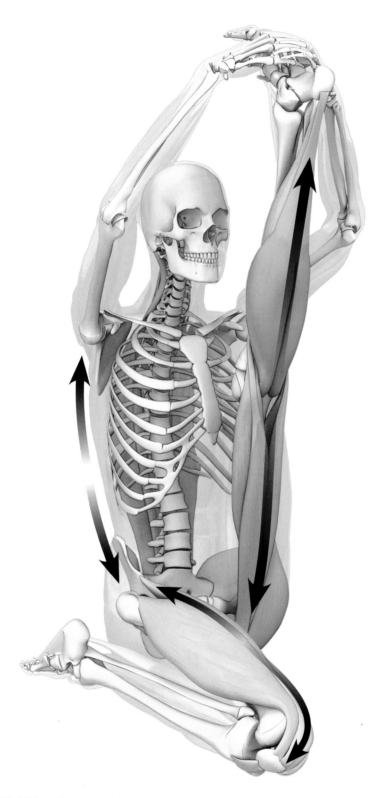

SUMMARY These combined actions orchestrate a linked stretch of the posterior kinetic chain. Use triangulation to locate the focal point of the pose. The knee extends and the hip flexes to stretch the hamstrings. Flexing the trunk stretches the erector spinae and quadratus lumborum and draws the back of the pelvis up, creating a further pull on the hamstrings at their attachments on the sitting bones. Flexing the hip stretches the gluteus maximus.

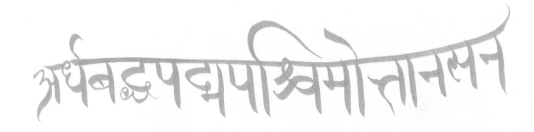

ARDHA BADHA PADMA PASCHIMOTTANASANA

HALF-BOUND LOTUS FORWARD FOLD

ARDHA BADHA PADMA PASCHIMOTTANASANA HAS TWO PARALLEL STORIES—A forward bend and a hip opener. The straight-leg hip flexes and the knee extends, with the trunk folding forward. The bent-leg hip flexes, abducts, and externally rotates, with the foot placed into Lotus (Padmasana) position, thus opening the hip. If you can't put the foot into Lotus, use a less difficult placement of the bent leg, for example, Janu Sirsasana. One arm reaches behind the back and grasps the big toe of the Lotus foot; the other hand grasps the outside of the straight-leg foot. It is important to note that you must have length in the internal rotators of the bent-knee hip in order to externally rotate it and place the foot on the thigh. Never force the foot into Padmasana position, as you can injure the knee. If you are unfamiliar with this concept, review the section on Lotus (page 96). Use facilitated stretching of the internal rotators to dissolve blockages, so that you can eventually place the foot easily into Padmasana.

BASIC JOINT POSITIONS

- The straight-leg hip flexes.
- The knee extends.
- The ankle plantar flexes.
- The foot everts.
- The bent-leg hip flexes, abducts, and externally rotates.
- The ankle plantar flexes.
- The foot everts.

- The trunk flexes.
- The front-arm shoulder flexes, abducts, and externally rotates.
- The back-arm shoulder extends, adducts, and internally rotates.
- The elbows flex.
- The forward wrist flexes.
- The back wrist extends.

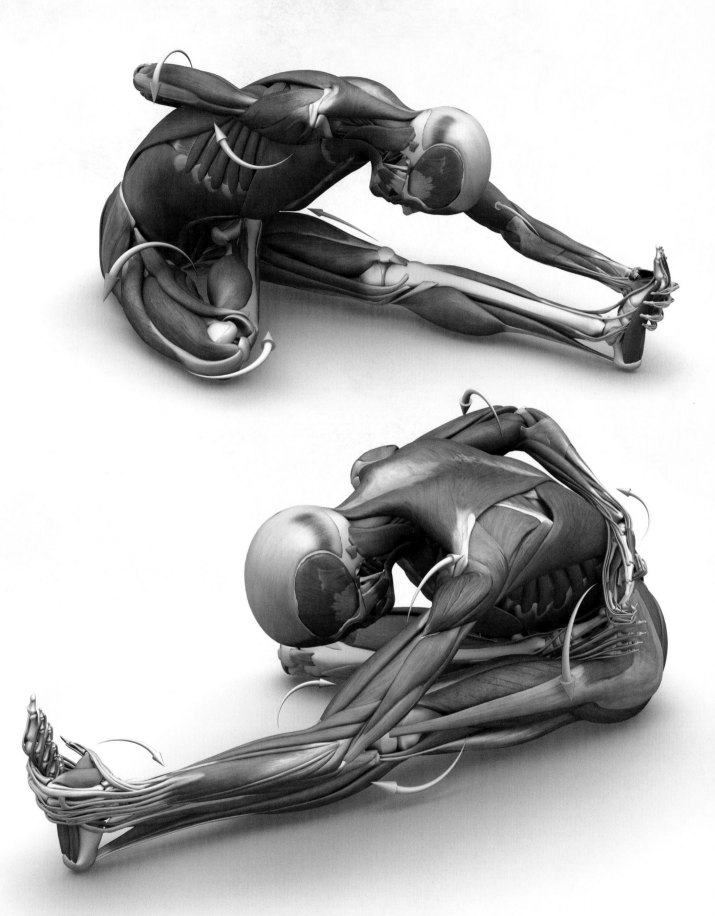

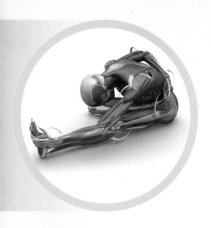

Ardha Badha Padma
Paschimottanasana Preparation

Cradle the leg that is to be placed in Lotus in the arms, as shown. Holding the knee in the crook of the elbow stabilizes it. Take care to maintain the knee joint as a hinge. Do not allow the knee to sag forward, as this can create joint incongruency, potentially injuring the cartilage or stretching the lateral collateral ligament of the knee.

Next, place the foot into Padmasana on the opposite hip. If you're unable to safely obtain Padmasana, position the leg in Janu Sirsasana. Grasp the straight-leg foot with a belt or rope, and flex the elbows to draw the body forward. Initially bend the straight-leg knee, as with the other forward bends.

Once you are comfortable in this position, move toward the final variation of the pose. Use a belt to grasp the Lotus foot with the hand behind the back. Have another belt around the straight-leg foot. Bend the elbow of the forward arm to draw the body over the leg. At the same time, pull away from the back with the arm that is holding the Lotus foot. Notice how these actions draw the body deeper into the pose, stabilizing it. Work toward grasping both feet with the hands.

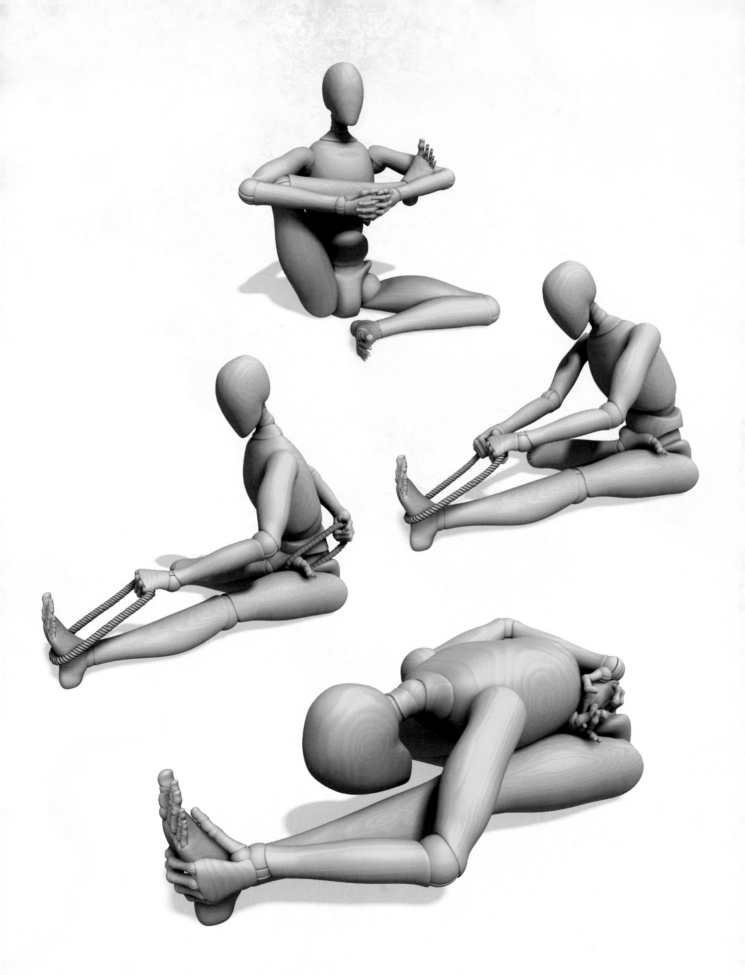

ARDHA BADHA PADMA PASCHIMOTTANASANA—HALF-BOUND LOTUS FORWARD FOLD **147**

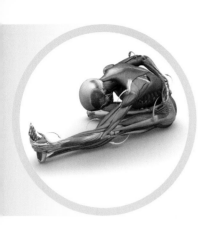

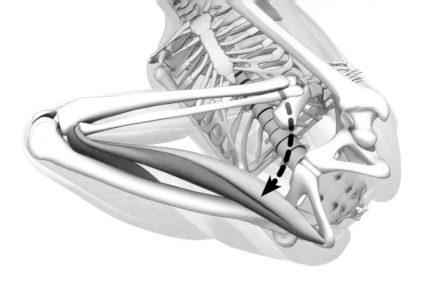

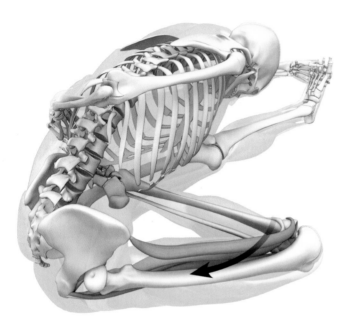

STEP 1 Flex, abduct, and externally rotate the bent-leg thigh. This contracts the sartorius. Activate the hamstrings to flex the knee. The knee is not a pure hinge joint; it allows for some rotation. Use this principle to protect the knee joint surfaces in this pose. Press down on the lower side of the Padmasana foot to preferentially activate the outer-side hamstrings. Because these muscles insert on the fibula bone at the outside of the lower leg, engaging them with this cue externally rotates the lower leg at the knee and moves the joint toward congruency.

▶ **STEP 2** Abduct and externally rotate the hip of the bent leg. Contract the deep external rotator muscles of the hip by tucking the tailbone under. Engage the gluteus medius and tensor fascia lata to draw the knee toward the floor.

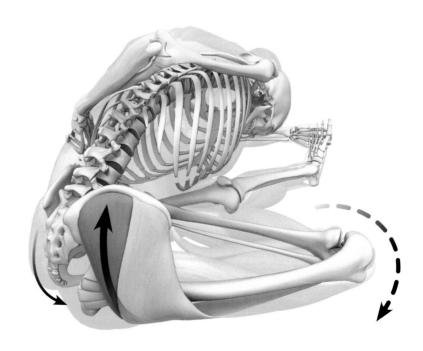

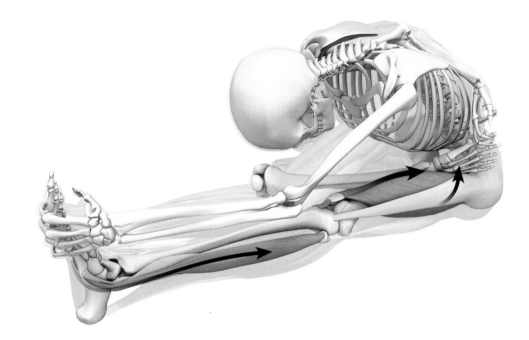

▲ STEP 3 Contract the quadriceps to straighten the knee of the extended leg. Engage the tensor fascia lata to flex and internally rotate the hip as well as stabilize the outer side of the knee. This exemplifies how a polyarticular muscle—one that crosses multiple joints—can be used to create multiple actions. In this case, the tensor fascia lata flexes the hip and extends the knee. The gluteus minimus (hidden under the tensor fascia lata) synergizes hip flexion and internal rotation. Use the peronei on the outside of the lower leg to evert the ankle and open the sole of the foot. Balance this eversion with an inversion force by engaging the tibialis posterior muscle, stabilizing the ankle.

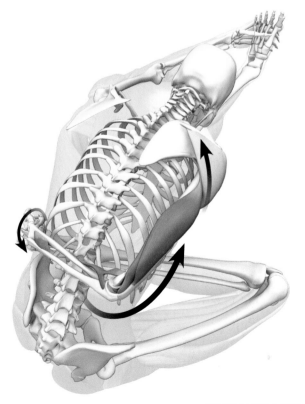

STEP 4 If you're able to grasp the foot with the arm behind the back, then pronate the forearm as if you are attempting to turn the palm downward, and lock the grip on the foot. This creates a "wringing" effect from the wrist to the elbow. Then activate the triceps to pull backward on the big toe and foot, generating a force that draws the shoulder and elbow back and rotates the chest away from the straight leg.

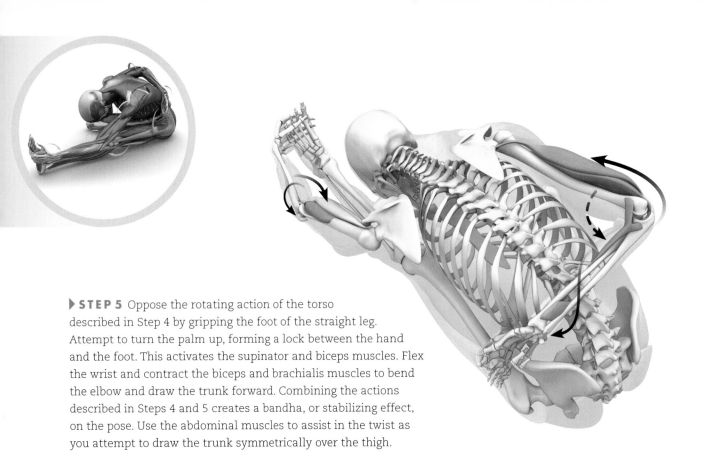

▶ **STEP 5** Oppose the rotating action of the torso described in Step 4 by gripping the foot of the straight leg. Attempt to turn the palm up, forming a lock between the hand and the foot. This activates the supinator and biceps muscles. Flex the wrist and contract the biceps and brachialis muscles to bend the elbow and draw the trunk forward. Combining the actions described in Steps 4 and 5 creates a bandha, or stabilizing effect, on the pose. Use the abdominal muscles to assist in the twist as you attempt to draw the trunk symmetrically over the thigh.

STEP 6 Internally rotate the arm that is reaching behind the back by engaging the subscapularis, teres major, latissimus dorsi, and pectoralis major. A cue for contracting these muscles is to attempt to lift the hand away from the back.

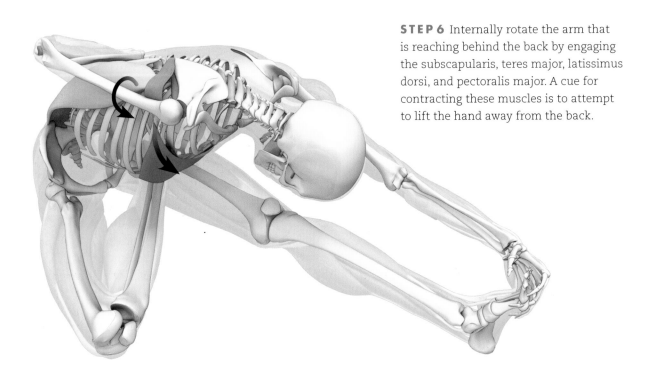

▶ **STEP 7** Activate the latissimus dorsi of the arm that is grasping the straight-leg foot. Imagine doing a chin-up to engage this muscle. See how this draws the trunk deeper into the forward bend.

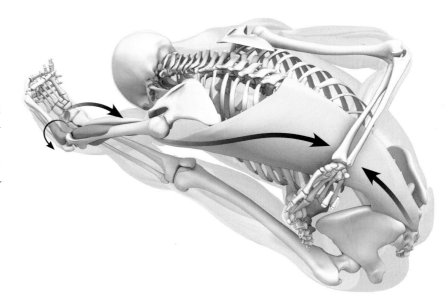

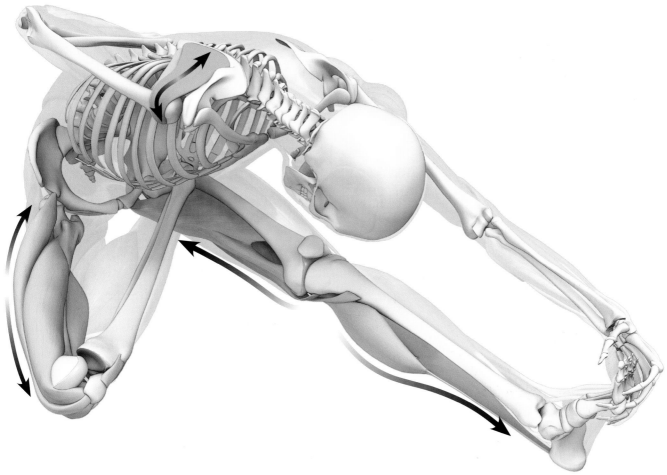

SUMMARY All of these actions combine to stretch the bent-leg quadriceps, the erector spinae, and the quadratus lumborum muscles of the back. The straight-leg gluteus maximus, hamstrings, and gastrocnemius all stretch as well. Internally rotating the shoulder lengthens the infraspinatus and teres minor muscles. Placing one leg into Lotus or Padmasana position externally rotates the hip and stretches the tensor fascia lata and gluteus medius, which are internal rotators of the hip. These muscles also eccentrically contract to abduct the knee to the side.

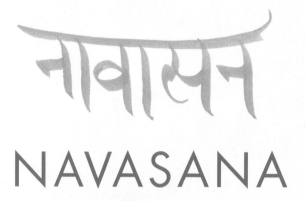

नावासन

NAVASANA

BOAT POSE

I PLACE NAVASANA IN THE FORWARD-FOLDING SECTION BECAUSE IT FLEXES the trunk. This is a forward bend that requires constant muscular effort to maintain. For this reason, the main story in the pose is an isolated strengthening of the core abdominal muscles and not so much a focused stretch, as with the other forward bends. Moving outward from the abdominals, a number of steps can be taken to stabilize the pose. For example, squeezing the knees together isolates and engages the adductor muscles of the thighs. Contracting the quadriceps straightens the knees and engaging the psoas muscles flexes the hips. Similar subplots exist in the arms and shoulders. This type of co-activation produces the phenomenon of recruitment. For example, note that if you squeeze the knees together, you can more forcefully engage the abdominals.

BASIC JOINT POSITIONS

- The hips flex.
- The knees extend.
- The ankles plantar flex.
- The feet evert.

- The trunk flexes.
- The shoulders flex, adduct, and externally rotate.
- The forearms are neutral.

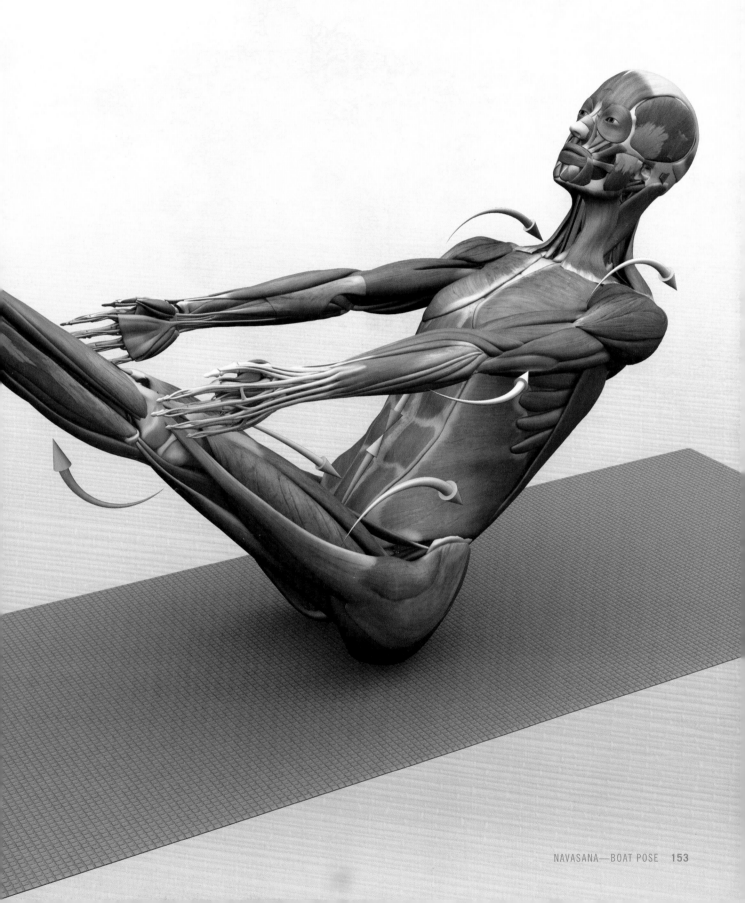

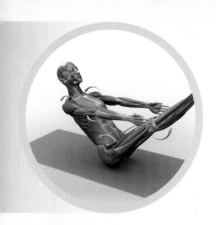

Navasana Preparation

Begin with the knees bent, and flex the hips. Hold the backs of the thighs with the hands to support the legs. Get a feel for squeezing the knees together. Activate the hip flexors and tense the abdominals. Then straighten the knees. Finally, extend the arms and arch the back slightly to take the full pose. If you're unable to achieve the full posture, use one of the intermediate variations shown. As you gain strength, work toward the classical variation of Navasana.

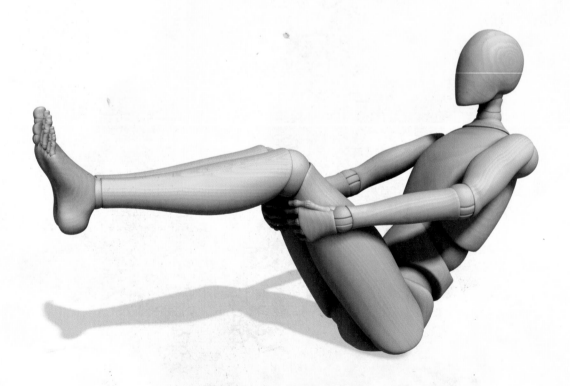

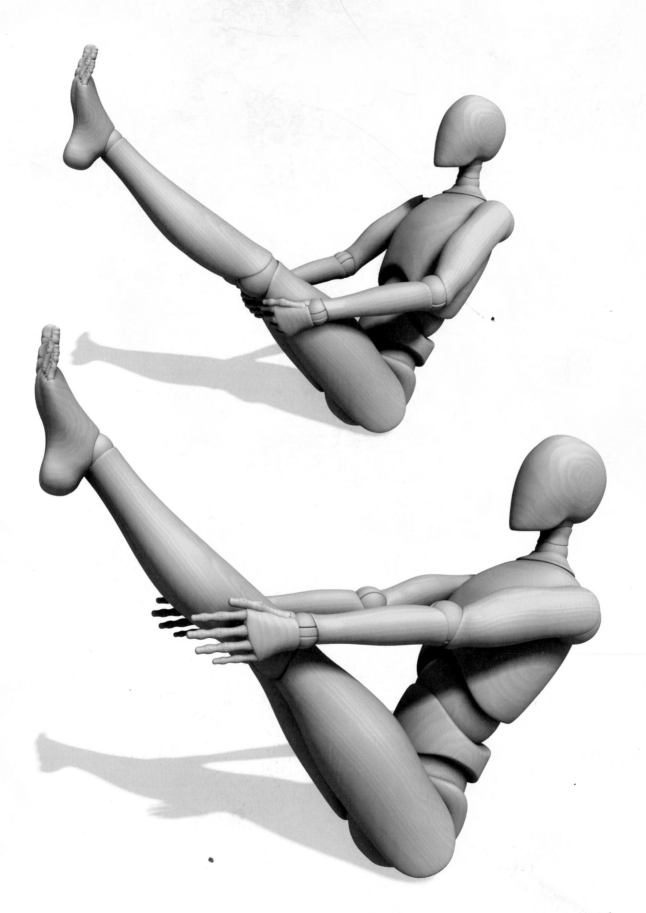

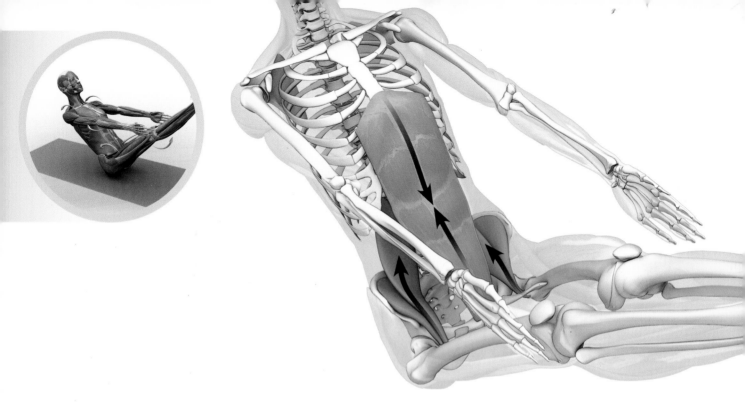

STEP 1 Contract the rectus abdominis at the front of the abdomen. In fact, you will activate all layers of the abdominals when you do this, including the transversus abdominis and both of the oblique abdominals. This is fine. They all flex the trunk. The psoas and its synergists, the pectineus and adductors longus and brevis, activate to flex the hips and draw the legs up. To feel the psoas engage, bend the knees with the feet on the ground and place your hands on the thighs. Resist with the hands while you attempt to draw the knees toward the chest. Look for this same feeling while in the full pose.

People tend to round the back in Navasana because they rely almost entirely on the abdominals to flex the trunk. Engaging the psoas flexes the hips and tilts the pelvis forward. The psoas major draws the lumbar spine forward into lordosis; this counteracts some of the lower back rounding caused by engaging the abdominals. It is important to combine both the psoas and the abdominal muscles to obtain the optimal form of the pose.

STEP 2 Activate the quadriceps to straighten the knees. Synergize the action of the quadriceps by engaging the tensor fascia lata. A cue for this is to place the hands on the outsides of the legs and try to draw them apart (abduct). Isolating the tensor fascia lata and gluteus medius has the added benefit of internally rotating the thighs. Contracting these muscles counteracts the external rotation component of the psoas and turns the kneecaps to face upward.

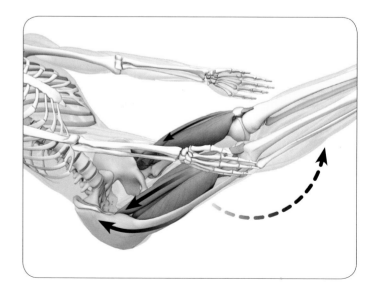

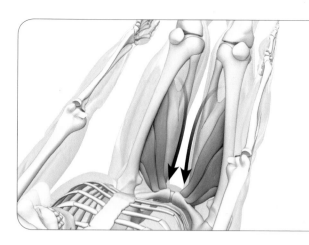

STEP 3 Squeeze the knees together to engage the adductor group. Note that the more anterior of these muscles, the adductors longus and brevis, also have fibers that externally rotate the thighs. This action is countered by the tensor fascia lata, as described in Step 2.

▶ **STEP 4** Arch the back to engage the erector spinae and quadratus lumborum. The quadratus lumborum acts synergistically with the psoas major to support the lumbar spine.

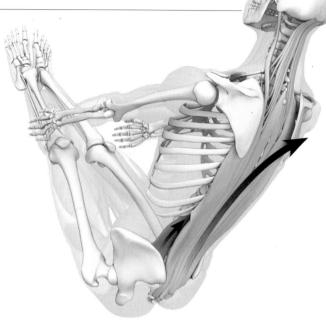

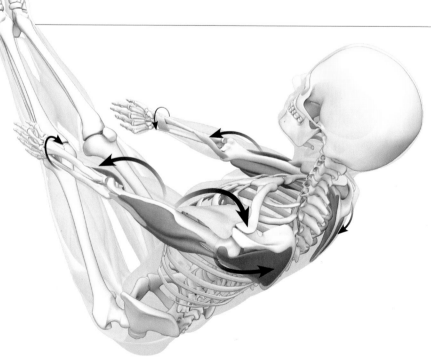

STEP 5 Extend the elbows by contracting the triceps. Use the pronators teres and quadratus to turn the forearms until the palms face the outer thighs. Activate the infraspinatus and teres minor muscles to turn the upper arms outward. This produces a helical "wringing" effect from the hands to the shoulders, stabilizing the elbows. Engage the anterior deltoids to lift the arms parallel to the floor.

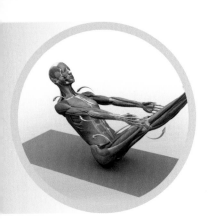

STEP 6 The rhomboids draw the shoulder blades toward the midline and stabilize them, opening the front of the chest. Once the scapulae are constrained in this position, contract the pectoralis minor and serratus anterior to expand and lift the ribcage. A cue for engaging these muscles is to hold the shoulder blades back and then attempt to roll the shoulders forward. The shoulders won't move but the contractile force of the pectoralis minor and serratus anterior is transmuted to the ribcage, lifting it upwards as shown.

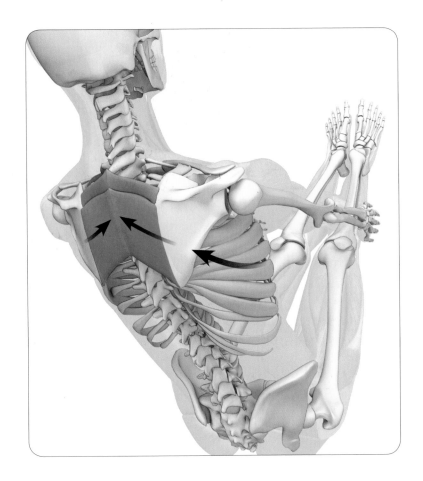

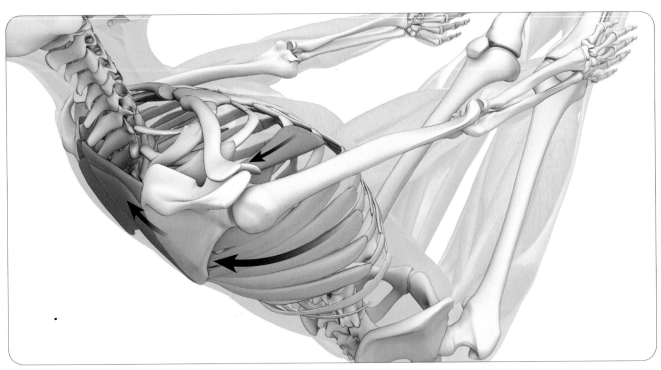

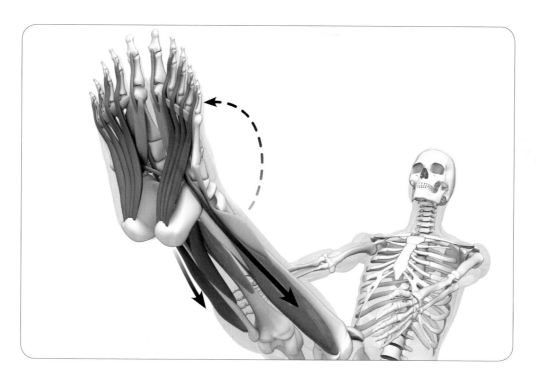

▲ **STEP 7** Plantar flex the ankles to point the feet. This activates the gastrocnemius/soleus muscles of the calves (not shown). These muscles connect to the heel via the Achilles tendon. Use the peroneus longus and brevis muscles on the sides of the lower legs to evert the ankles, turning the feet outward and opening the soles. Balance this action by engaging the tibialis posterior, which spans the tibia and fibula bones of the lower legs. The tibialis posterior inverts the foot and dynamizes the arch. Co-contract the peronei and tibialis posterior to stabilize the ankle joints. Flex (point) the toes using the extrinsic toe flexors (those originating from the lower legs) and the intrinsic toe flexors (those originating from the feet themselves).

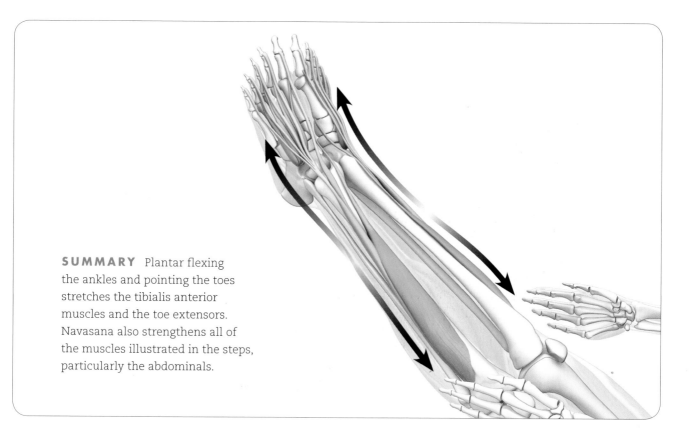

SUMMARY Plantar flexing the ankles and pointing the toes stretches the tibialis anterior muscles and the toe extensors. Navasana also strengthens all of the muscles illustrated in the steps, particularly the abdominals.

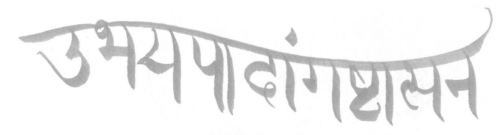

UBHAYA PADANGUSTHASANA

BOTH FEET BIG-TOE POSE

UBHAYA PADANGUSTHASANA ENGAGES MANY OF THE SAME MUSCLES AS Navasana. In addition, it links the upper and lower extremities, connecting the shoulder girdle with the pelvic girdle via the torso. Lifting the arms or bending the elbows accentuates flexing the hips and extending the knees. This creates a greater stretch of the backs of the legs, which is the focal point of this story. The grip on the big toes is an essential component, with the big toes flexing against the fingers and thumbs to create a lock. Ubhaya Padangusthasana is also a balancing pose, meaning that you can apply the principles of physics to stabilize the posture. For example, if you start to fall back, simply bend the knees to re-establish balance by lowering the center of gravity.

BASIC JOINT POSITIONS

- The hips flex.
- The knees extend.
- The ankles plantar flex.
- The feet evert.
- The trunk flexes.
- The shoulders flex, adduct, and externally rotate.
- The elbows extend.
- The forearms supinate.

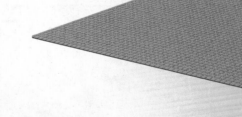

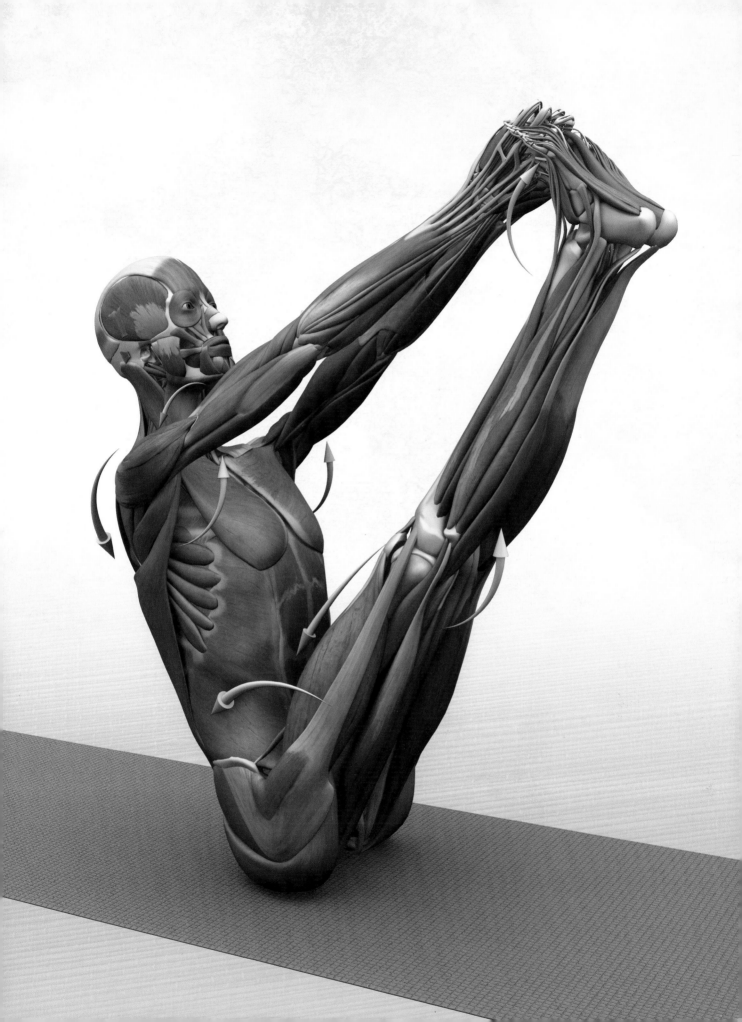

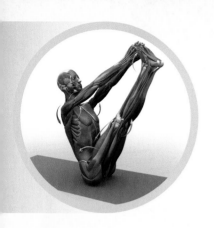

Ubhaya Padangusthasana
Preparation

Link the hands and feet with a belt. Keeping the feet together, bend the knees and allow them to fall outward to get a feel for balancing on the tailbone (coccyx) and ischial tuberosities. Do this a few times, holding for five to ten seconds (not more). Rest for several moments in-between to give the unconscious brain an opportunity to create the circuitry to balance more efficiently. Note that bending the knees lowers the center of gravity for a more stable pose. Note also how your balance improves with each successive repetition. Grasp the big toes with the thumb and first two fingers. Flex the wrists and bend the big toes to lock the grip. As your equilibrium improves, straighten the knees.

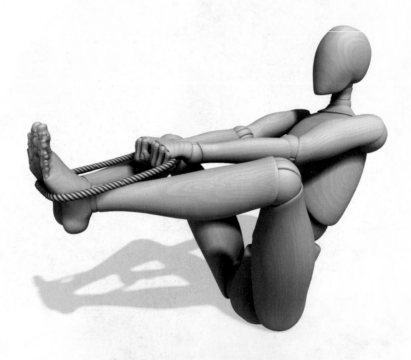

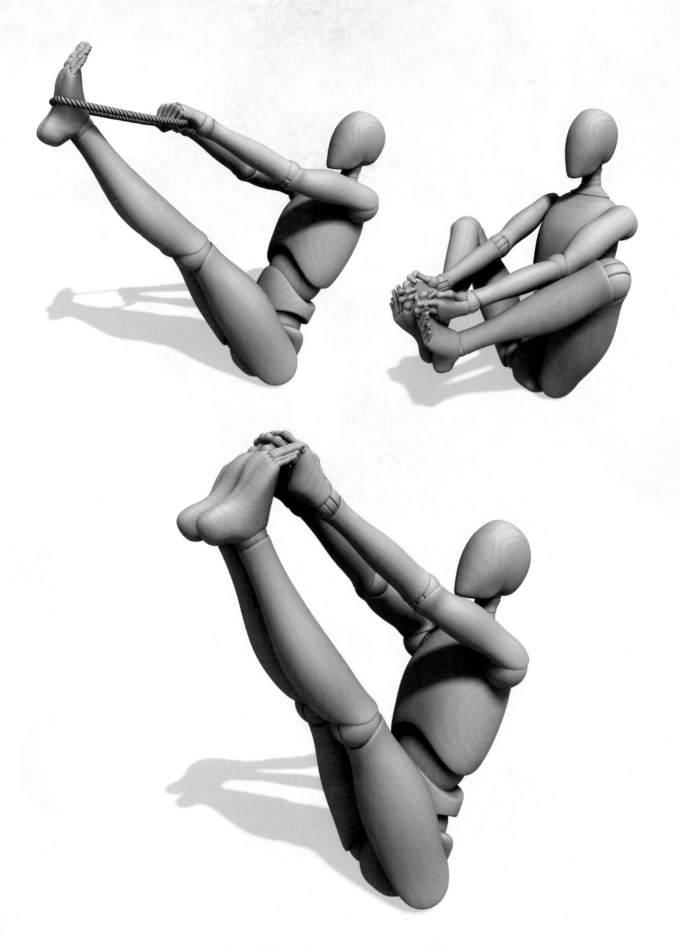

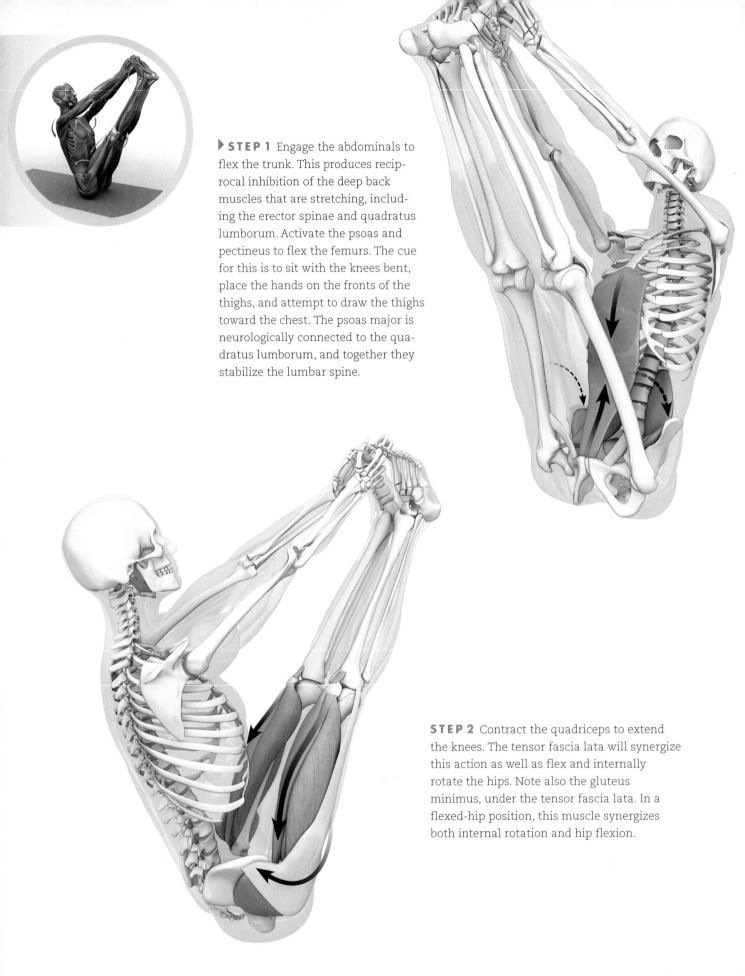

▶ **STEP 1** Engage the abdominals to flex the trunk. This produces reciprocal inhibition of the deep back muscles that are stretching, including the erector spinae and quadratus lumborum. Activate the psoas and pectineus to flex the femurs. The cue for this is to sit with the knees bent, place the hands on the fronts of the thighs, and attempt to draw the thighs toward the chest. The psoas major is neurologically connected to the quadratus lumborum, and together they stabilize the lumbar spine.

STEP 2 Contract the quadriceps to extend the knees. The tensor fascia lata will synergize this action as well as flex and internally rotate the hips. Note also the gluteus minimus, under the tensor fascia lata. In a flexed-hip position, this muscle synergizes both internal rotation and hip flexion.

STEP 3 Squeeze the knees together with the adductor group. As discussed in Navasana, the more anterior of these muscles externally rotate the thighs. Balance this action by engaging the tensor fascia lata and gluteus minimus, as described above. The cue for this is to attempt to draw the legs apart while holding the feet together, internally rotating the legs and bringing the kneecaps to face straight up in a neutral position.

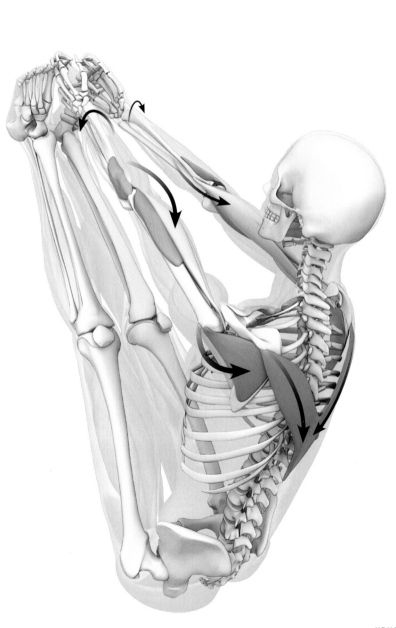

STEP 4 Grip the toes and turn the forearm bones so that the elbow creases begin to face upward. This aids to lock the grip of the hands. Bend the elbows by contracting the biceps and brachialis muscles. Note how this draws the trunk toward the thighs and the feet toward the head. Engage the infraspinatus and teres minor muscles of the rotator cuff to externally rotate the shoulders. Grip the big toes firmly and attempt to drag the hands upward, as if lifting the arms. Draw the elbows out to the sides. This engages the anterior and lateral portions of the deltoid muscles. The arms do not actually lift, but the trunk is drawn closer to the legs. Feel how this action augments the stretch at the backs of the legs.

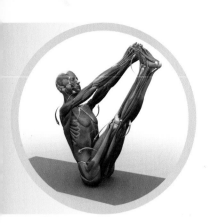

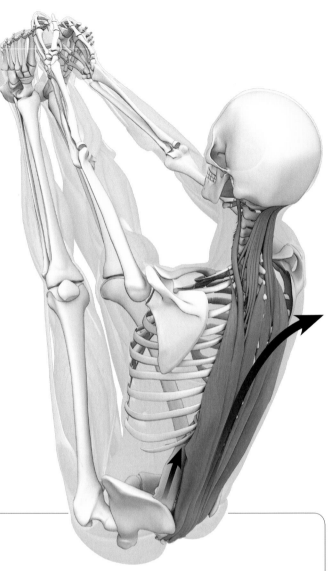

STEP 5 Arch the back by engaging the erector spinae and quadratus lumborum. Notice that, because the hands hold the feet, arching the back actually pulls the thighs closer to the chest. The quadratus lumborum also assists the psoas major in stabilizing the lumbar spine.

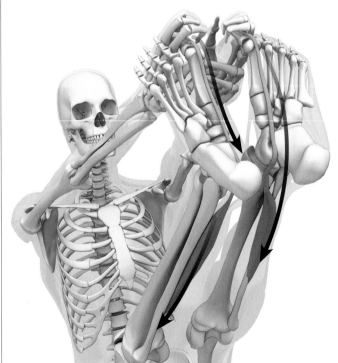

STEP 6 Activate the flexors hallucis longus and brevis to flex the big toes and grip the fingers, as shown here.

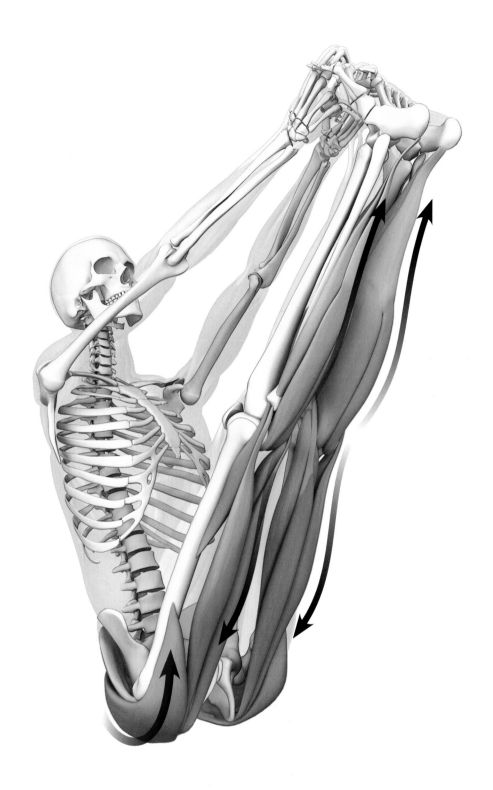

SUMMARY These various subplots work together toward a central theme—the stretch of the muscles at the backs of the legs, including the gastrocnemius/soleus complex, hamstrings, adductor magnus, and gluteus maximus. There is also a stretch of the deep back muscles, which eccentrically contract to arch the back, as described in Step 5.

RESTORATIVE POSES
VIPARITA KARANI LEGS-UP-THE-WALL POSE

Relax the body in Viparita Karani. This pose gently extends the back to balance the muscles that were stretched in the forward bends. It is also a mild inversion, with beneficial effects on the cardiovascular system, including a temporary lowering of heart rate and blood pressure.

Place a block between the wall and the bolster and then tilt the pelvis onto the block, with the small of the back draped over the bolster. Use a blanket under the head to keep the neck slightly flexed. Let the arms fall out to the sides with the palms facing up.

You can also use a chair variation for this pose. Flexing the knees relaxes the hamstrings. Flexing the hips relaxes the psoas and its synergists. Stay in the pose for five minutes or more to prepare for Savasana.

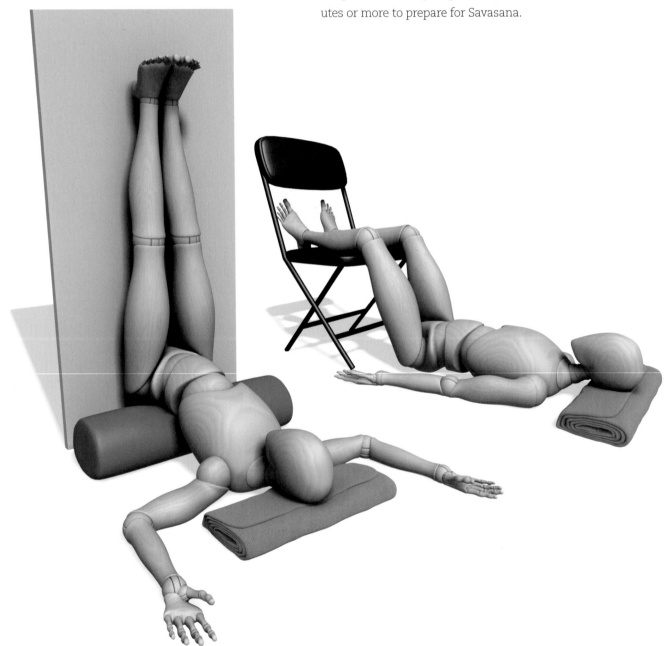

SAVASANA CORPSE POSE

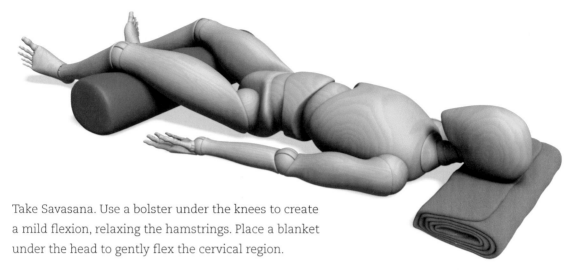

Take Savasana. Use a bolster under the knees to create a mild flexion, relaxing the hamstrings. Place a blanket under the head to gently flex the cervical region.

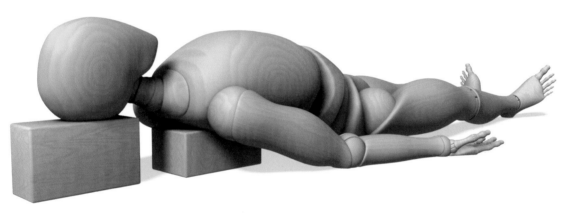

Alternatively, place a block in the region of the shoulder blades to passively stretch the intercostal muscles and expand the chest. Avoid extending the neck as this tightens the throat and can harm the cervical spine region. Instead use a block under the head to gently flex the neck.

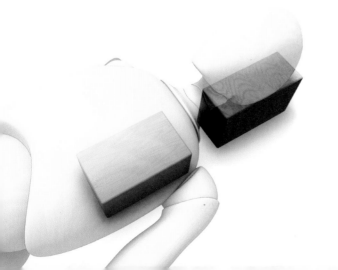

This image illustrates the orientation of the blocks and proper placement under the body.

Allow the feet to fall out to the sides and the palms to turn upward. Close the eyes and rest in Savasana for five to ten minutes to complete your practice.

MOVEMENT INDEX

MOVEMENT INDEX

Movements of the body have specific names. It is important to learn these names, both for teaching others yoga and for analyzing the muscles that produce the positions of the body. As a yoga teacher, it is always better to communicate your instructions in terminology that students can easily understand. Know the scientific names of the movements and have clear explanations to describe the movements in layperson's terms. Make your instructions as precise and uncomplicated as you can.

Remember that muscles contract to position the joints and appendages in the pose. If you know the joint positions, you can analyze which muscles to engage to produce the asana. With this knowledge comes the ability to use precise cues to communicate how to sculpt and stabilize the body in the pose, stretch the correct muscles, and create bandhas. Thus, unlocking the asana begins with a clear understanding of body movements.

There are six basic movements of the body: Flexion, Extension, Adduction, Abduction, Internal Rotation, and External Rotation. These movements take place in three planes, as shown here. The anatomic position is the reference point to define the direction of movement.

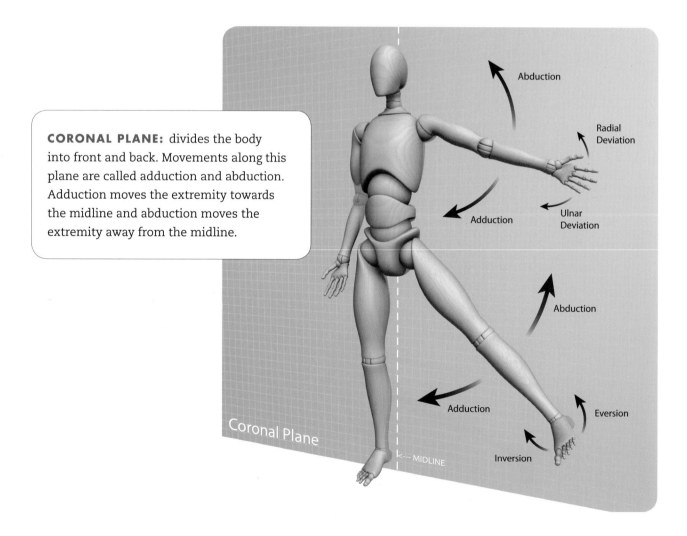

CORONAL PLANE: divides the body into front and back. Movements along this plane are called adduction and abduction. Adduction moves the extremity towards the midline and abduction moves the extremity away from the midline.

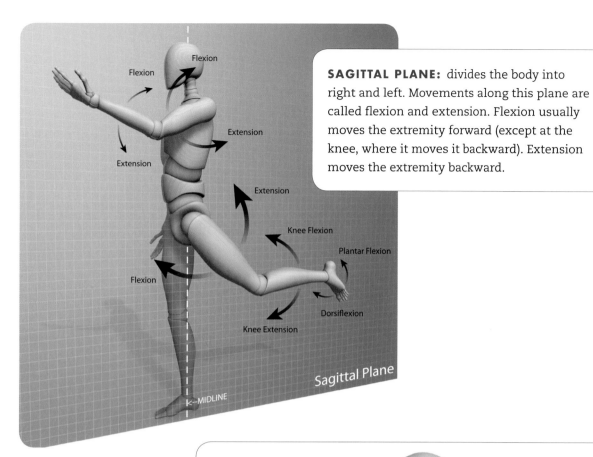

SAGITTAL PLANE: divides the body into right and left. Movements along this plane are called flexion and extension. Flexion usually moves the extremity forward (except at the knee, where it moves it backward). Extension moves the extremity backward.

TRANSVERSE PLANE: divides the body into upper and lower halves. Movement along this plane is called rotation. Rotation is further classified as internal (towards the midline) and external (away from the midline). Internal and external rotation are also referred to as medial and lateral rotation, respectively.

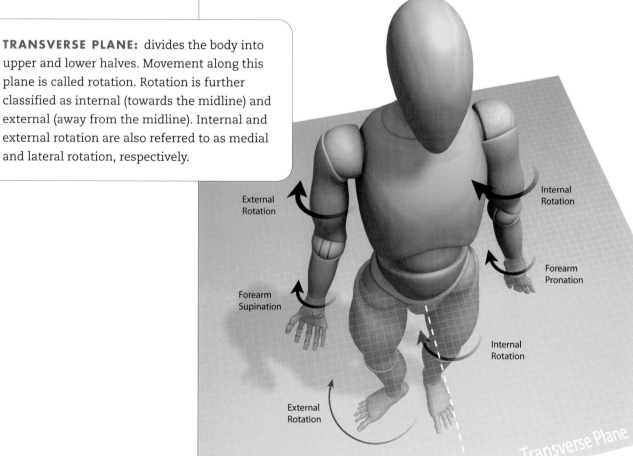

MOVEMENT INDEX

Krounchasana and Parighasana are presented as examples of how to analyze the basic joint positions in a yoga pose. The order represents the sequence of movements that create the form of the pose.

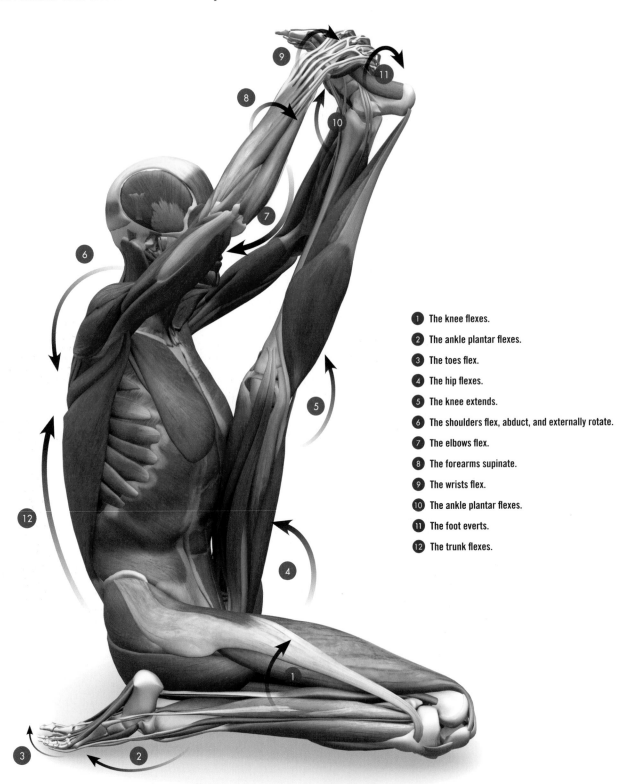

1. The knee flexes.
2. The ankle plantar flexes.
3. The toes flex.
4. The hip flexes.
5. The knee extends.
6. The shoulders flex, abduct, and externally rotate.
7. The elbows flex.
8. The forearms supinate.
9. The wrists flex.
10. The ankle plantar flexes.
11. The foot everts.
12. The trunk flexes.

1 The knee flexes.

2 The ankle plantar flexes.

3 The toes flex.

4 The hip flexes.

5 The knee extends.

6 The ankle plantar flexes.

7 The trunk laterally flexes.

8 The shoulders flex, abduct, and externally rotate.

9 The elbows extend.

10 The forearms pronate.

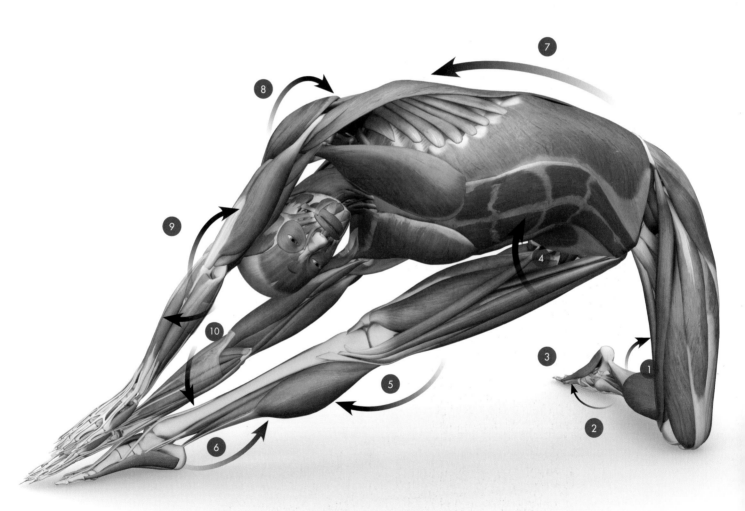

MOVEMENT TABLES

Neck

Muscle	Flexion	Extension	Lateral Flexion	Lateral Extension	Rotation
Semispinalis capitis		●	●	●	●
Splenius capitis		●	●	●	●
Sternocleidomastoid	●		●	●	●
Levator scapulae		●	●	●	
Trapezius		●	●	●	●

Trunk

Muscle	Flexion	Extension	Lateral Flexion	Rotation
External oblique	●		●	●
Internal oblique	●		●	●
Rectus abdominis	●			
Spinalis thoracis		●		
Lateral intertransversi			●	
Interspinales		●		
Longissimus thoracis		●		
Iliocostalis lumborum		●		
Multifidus		●		
Rotatores		●		●
Quadratus lumborum		●	●	
Psoas major	●		●	
Iliacus	●		●	

Hip

Muscle	Flexion	Extension	Adduction	Abduction	Internal Rotation	External Rotation
Gluteus maximus		●				●
Gluteus medius	●	●		●	●	●
Gluteus minimus	●	●		●	●	●
Tensor fascia lata	●			●	●	
Psoas major	●					●
Iliacus	●					●
Rectus femoris	●			●		
Sartorius	●			●		●
Pectineus	●		●			●
Adductor magnus		●	●			●
Adductor longus	●		●			●
Adductor brevis	●		●			●
Gracilis	●		●			●
Piriformis				●		●
Gemellus superior				●		●
Gemellus inferior				●		●
Obturator internus				●		●
Obturator externus						●
Quadratus femoris			●			●
Semitendinosus		●			●	
Semimembranosus		●			●	
Biceps femoris		●				●

MOVEMENT TABLES

Knee

Muscle	Flexion	Extension	Internal Rotation	External Rotation
Vastus medialis		●		
Vastus lateralis		●		
Vastus intermedius		●		
Rectus femoris		●		
Sartorius	●			●
Semitendinosus	●		●	
Semimembranosus	●		●	
Biceps femoris	●			●
Gracilis	●		●	
Popliteus	●			
Gastrocnemius	●			

Lower Leg

Muscle	Ankle Plantar Flexion	Ankle Dorsiflexion	Foot Eversion	Foot Inversion	Toe Flexion	Toe Extension
Gastrocnemius	●					
Soleus	●					
Tibialis anterior		●		●		
Tibialis posterior	●			●		
Peroneus longus	●		●			
Peroneus brevis	●		●			
Peroneus tertius	●		●			
Flexor digitorum longus	●			●	●	
Flexor hallucis longus	●			●	●	
Extensor digitorum longus		●	●			●
Extensor hallucis longus		●		●		●

Foot

Muscle	Toe Flexion	Toe Extension	Toe Adduction	Toe Abduction
Flexor digitorum brevis	●			
Flexor hallucis brevis	●			
Flexor digiti minimi brevis	●			
Extensor digitorum brevis		●		
Extensor hallucis brevis		●		
Abductor digiti minimi				●
Abductor hallucis				●
Adductor hallucis			●	
Lumbricales	●	●	●	
Plantar interosseus	●		●	
Dorsal interosseus	●			●

Hand

Muscle	Flexion	Extension	Adduction	Abduction
Flexor digitorum superficialis	●			
Flexor digitorum profundus	●			
Flexor pollicis longus	●			
Flexor pollicis brevis	●			
Flexor digiti minimi brevis	●			
Extensor digitorum		●		
Extensor pollicis longus		●		
Extensor pollicis brevis		●		
Extensor indicis		●		
Extensor digiti minimi		●		
Abductor pollicis longus				●
Abductor pollicis brevis				●
Adductor pollicis			●	
Abductor digiti minimi				●
Lumbricales	●	●		
Dorsal interosseus	●	●	●	

MOVEMENT TABLES

Arm and Wrist

Muscle	Elbow Flexion	Elbow Extension	Forearm Pronation	Forearm Supination	Wrist Flexion	Wrist Extension	Wrist Ulnar Deviation	Wrist Radial Deviation
Biceps brachii	●			●				
Brachialis	●							
Triceps brachii		●						
Anconeus		●						
Brachioradialis	●							
Supinator				●				
Pronator teres			●					
Pronator quadratus			●					
Extensor carpi radialis longus						●		●
Extensor carpi radialis brevis						●		●
Extensor carpi ulnaris						●	●	
Flexor carpi radialis					●			●
Flexor carpi ulnaris					●		●	
Extensor digitorum						●		
Extensor pollicis brevis								●
Extensor pollicis longus				●				●
Abductor pollicis longus								●

Shoulder

Muscle	Retraction	Protraction	Elevation	Depression	Flexion	Extension	Adduction	Abduction	Internal Rotation	External Rotation
Rhomboids	●									
Serratus anterior		●	●					●		
Trapezius	●		●	●			●	●		
Levator scapulae		●	●							
Latissimus dorsi	●			●		●	●		●	
Teres major						●	●		●	
Pectoralis major				●	●		●		●	
Pectoralis minor		●		●						
Anterior deltoid					●				●	
Lateral deltoid								●		
Posterior deltoid						●				●
Supraspinatus								●		
Infraspinatus										●
Teres minor							●			●
Subscapularis									●	
Biceps brachii					●					
Coracobrachialis					●		●			
Triceps brachii						●	●			

ANATOMY
INDEX

ANATOMY INDEX
BONES

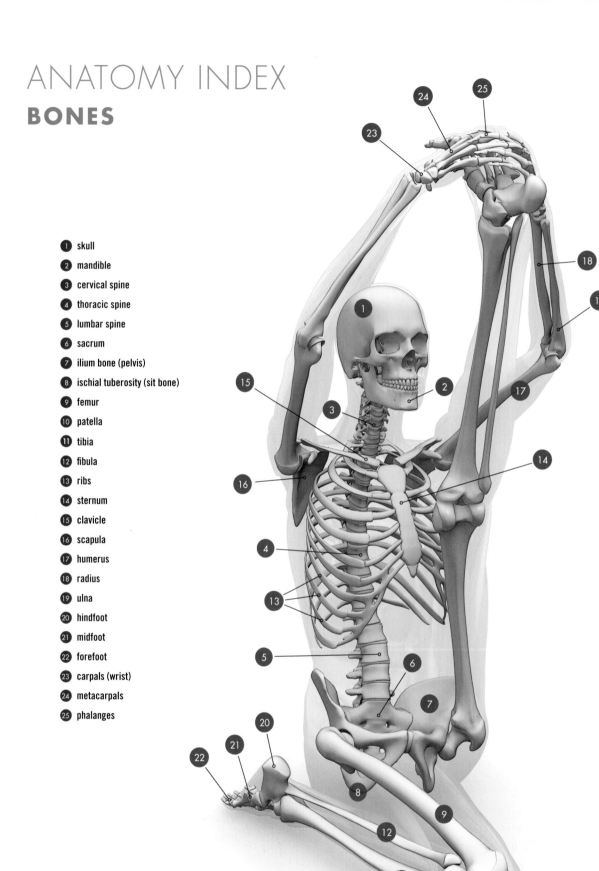

1. skull
2. mandible
3. cervical spine
4. thoracic spine
5. lumbar spine
6. sacrum
7. ilium bone (pelvis)
8. ischial tuberosity (sit bone)
9. femur
10. patella
11. tibia
12. fibula
13. ribs
14. sternum
15. clavicle
16. scapula
17. humerus
18. radius
19. ulna
20. hindfoot
21. midfoot
22. forefoot
23. carpals (wrist)
24. metacarpals
25. phalanges

AXIAL AND APPENDICULAR SKELETONS

AXIAL SKELETON

The axial skeleton is composed of the skull, spine, and ribcage. It links the upper and lower appendicular skeletons. Thus, the two subdivisions of the skeleton can be used to affect and influence each other.

For example, in Parighasana, connecting the hands to the straight-leg foot laterally flexes the trunk (axial skeleton).

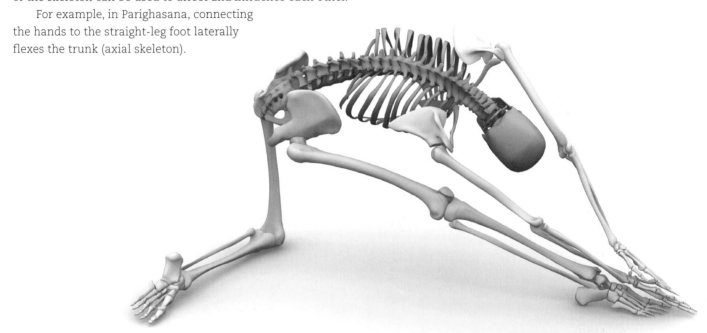

APPENDICULAR SKELETON

The upper appendicular skeleton is composed of the shoulder (pectoral) girdle and the upper extremities. The shoulder girdle, which is composed of the scapula and clavicle, connects the arm to the trunk and thereby links the upper appendicular skeleton to the axial skeleton.

The lower appendicular skeleton is composed of the pelvic girdle and lower extremities. The pelvic girdle is composed of the iliac bones, the ischia, the pubic bones, and the pubic symphysis. The pelvic girdle connects the lower extremities to the axial skeleton.

It is important to understand the subdivisions of the skeleton because the appendicular skeleton can be used to leverage and move the axial skeleton. Put another way, connecting the hand to the foot affects the spine.

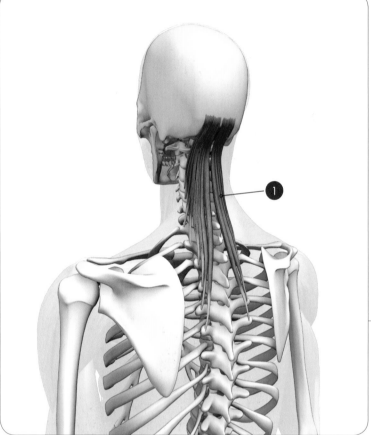

Legend

O = Origin. The proximal site where a muscle attaches to a bone.

I = Insertion. The distal site where a muscle attaches to a bone.

A = Action. The joint movement produced when the muscle contracts.

1 **Semispinalis capitis**
   O: Transverse processes of lower cervical and upper thoracic vertebrae.
   I: Occipital bone.
   A: Extends head (tilts it back), assists in turning head.

2 **Splenius capitis**
   O: Spinous processes of C7 and T1-4.
   I: Mastoid process of skull, behind ear.
   A: Extends head and neck; when one side contracts, laterally flexes neck; turns head toward side of individual muscle.

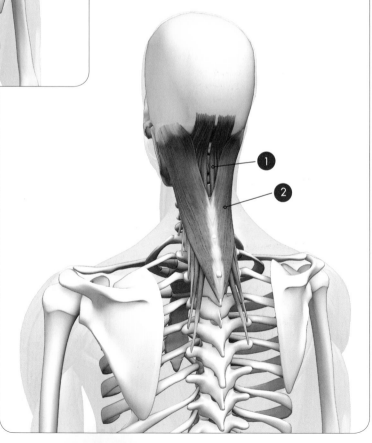

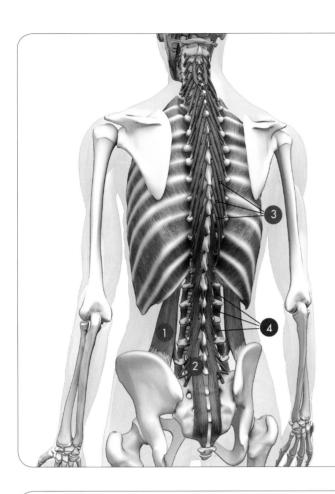

❶ Quadratus lumborum

O: Posterior (back) of iliac crest.

I: Back part of rib 12, transverse processes of L1-4.

A: Laterally flexes spine (bends to side); extends and stabilizes lumbar spine; stabilizes rib 12, drawing it down during deep inhalation.

❷ Multifidus

O: Back of sacrum and posterior superior iliac spine, transverse processes of lumbar, thoracic, and cervical vertebrae (all the way up the spine).

I: Two vertebrae above the vertebrae of origin; fibers are directed diagonally toward the midline and onto the spinous processes of the vertebrae of insertion.

A: Stabilizes spine during extension, flexion, and rotation.

❸ Semispinalis thoracis

O: Transverse processes of T6-10.

I: Spinous processes of lower cervical and upper thoracic vertebrae.

A: Extends and rotates upper thoracic and lower cervical spine.

❹ Lateral intertransversi

O: Transverse processes of lumbar vertebrae.

I: Transverse process of vertebrae immediately above vertebrae of origin.

A: Laterally flexes lumbar spine.

❶ Serratus posterior superior

O: Ligamentum nuchae and spinous processes of C7-T4.

I: Ribs 2-5 on upper border.

A: Expands back of chest during deep inhalation by lifting ribs (is an accessory muscle of breathing).

❷ Serratus posterior inferior

O: Spinous processes of T11-12, L1-3, thoracolumbar fascia.

I: Lower borders of ribs 9-12.

A: Stabilizes lower ribs during inhalation.

❸ Spinalis thoracis

O: Transverse processes of T6-10.

I: Spinous processes of C6-7, T1-4.

A: Extends upper thoracic and lower cervical spine.

❹ Longissimus thoracis

O: Posterior sacrum, spinous processes of T11-12, L1-5.

I: Transverse processes of T1-12, medial part of ribs 4-12.

A: Laterally flexes and extends spine, aids to expand chest during inhalation.

❺ Iliocostalis lumborum

O: Posterior sacrum.

I: Posterior part of ribs 7-12.

A: Laterally flexes and extends lumbar spine.

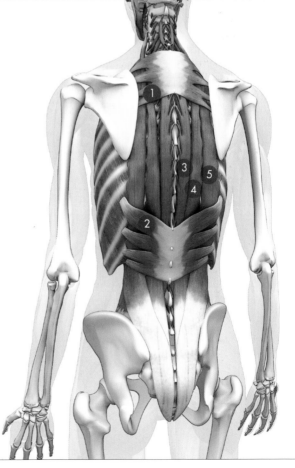

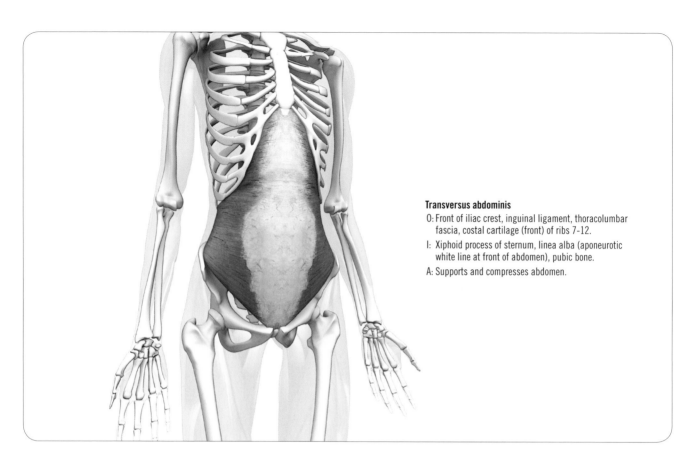

Transversus abdominis

O: Front of iliac crest, inguinal ligament, thoracolumbar fascia, costal cartilage (front) of ribs 7-12.

I: Xiphoid process of sternum, linea alba (aponeurotic white line at front of abdomen), pubic bone.

A: Supports and compresses abdomen.

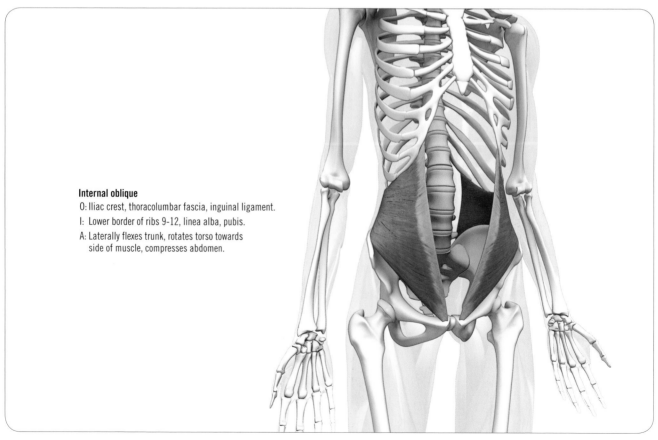

Internal oblique

O: Iliac crest, thoracolumbar fascia, inguinal ligament.

I: Lower border of ribs 9-12, linea alba, pubis.

A: Laterally flexes trunk, rotates torso towards side of muscle, compresses abdomen.

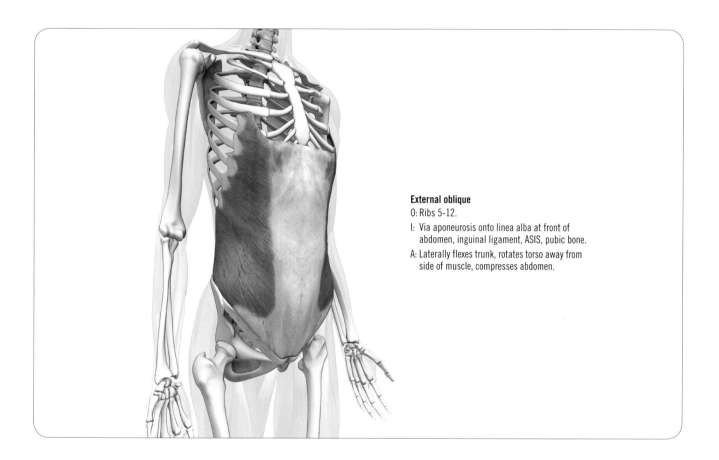

External oblique

O: Ribs 5-12.

I: Via aponeurosis onto linea alba at front of abdomen, inguinal ligament, ASIS, pubic bone.

A: Laterally flexes trunk, rotates torso away from side of muscle, compresses abdomen.

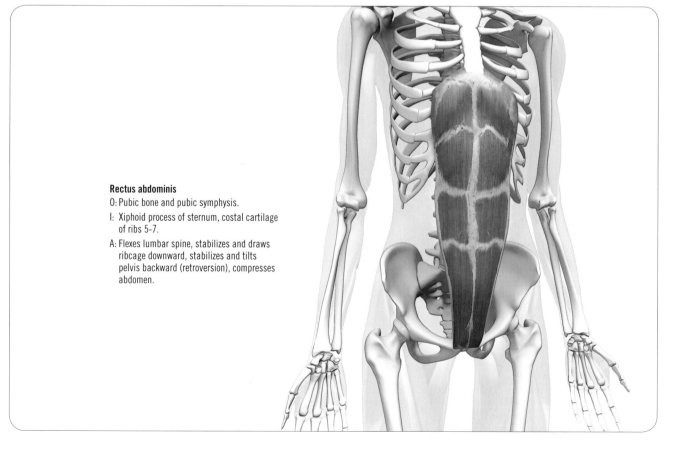

Rectus abdominis

O: Pubic bone and pubic symphysis.

I: Xiphoid process of sternum, costal cartilage of ribs 5-7.

A: Flexes lumbar spine, stabilizes and draws ribcage downward, stabilizes and tilts pelvis backward (retroversion), compresses abdomen.

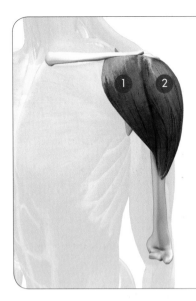

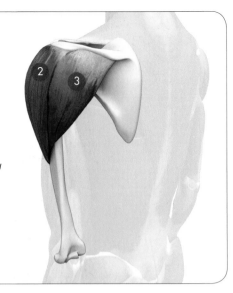

1 **Anterior deltoid**

O: Front and top of lateral third of clavicle.

I: Deltoid tuberosity on outer surface of humeral shaft.

A: Forward flexes and internally rotates humerus.

2 **Lateral deltoid**

O: Lateral border of acromion process of scapula.

I: Deltoid tuberosity on outer surface of humeral shaft.

A: Abducts humerus following initiation of movement by supraspinatus muscle of rotator cuff.

3 **Posterior deltoid**

O: Spine of scapula.

I: Deltoid tuberosity on outer surface of humeral shaft.

A: Extends and externally rotates humerus.

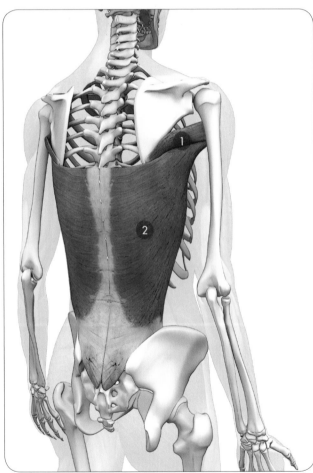

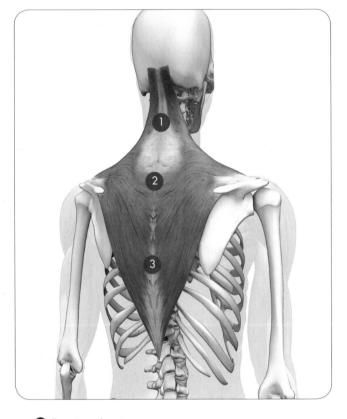

1 **Teres major**

O: Lower lateral border of scapula.

I: Bicipital groove of humerus.

A: Adducts and internally rotates humerus.

2 **Latissimus dorsi**

O: Thoracolumbar fascia, posterior portion of iliac crest, ribs 9-12, inferior border of scapula.

I: Bicipital groove of humerus.

A: Extends, adducts, and internally rotates humerus.

1 **Upper trapezius**

O: Occipital bone, ligamentum nuchae.

I: Upper border of spine of scapula.

A: Elevates (lifts) shoulder girdle, with lower trapezius rotates scapula to lift arm overhead.

2 **Middle trapezius**

O: Spinous processes of C7-T7.

I: Medial edge of acromion, posterior part of lateral third of clavicle.

A: Adducts (retracts) scapula.

3 **Lower trapezius**

O: Spinous processes of T8-12.

I: Medial edge of acromion, posterior part of lateral third of clavicle.

A: Depresses scapula, aids to hold body in arm balancing, with upper trapezius rotates scapula to lift arm overhead.

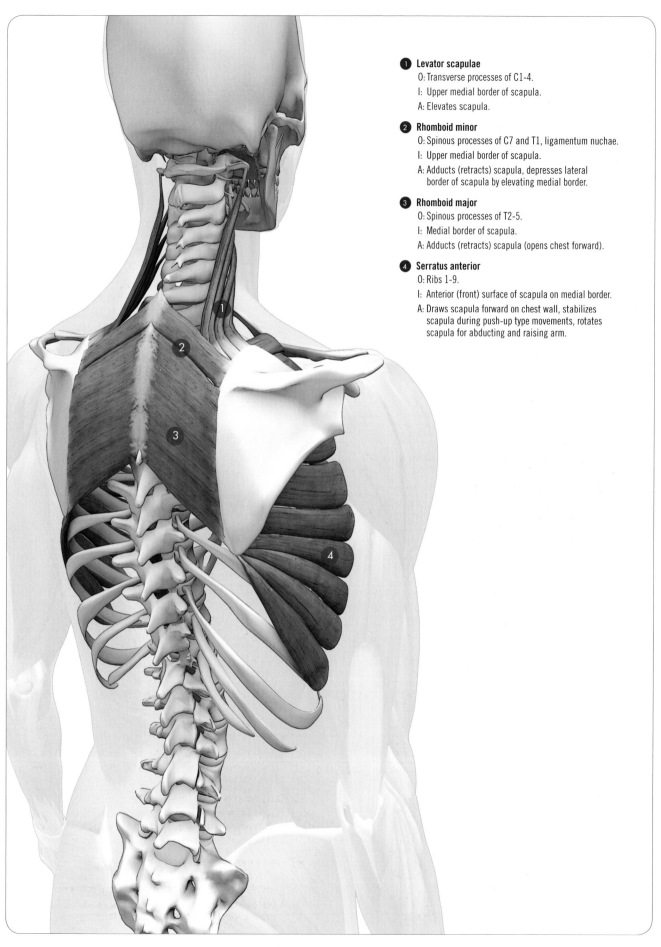

1 **Levator scapulae**

O: Transverse processes of C1-4.

I: Upper medial border of scapula.

A: Elevates scapula.

2 **Rhomboid minor**

O: Spinous processes of C7 and T1, ligamentum nuchae.

I: Upper medial border of scapula.

A: Adducts (retracts) scapula, depresses lateral border of scapula by elevating medial border.

3 **Rhomboid major**

O: Spinous processes of T2-5.

I: Medial border of scapula.

A: Adducts (retracts) scapula (opens chest forward).

4 **Serratus anterior**

O: Ribs 1-9.

I: Anterior (front) surface of scapula on medial border.

A: Draws scapula forward on chest wall, stabilizes scapula during push-up type movements, rotates scapula for abducting and raising arm.

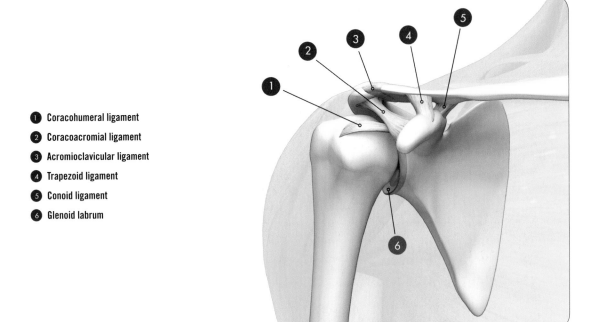

1. Coracohumeral ligament
2. Coracoacromial ligament
3. Acromioclavicular ligament
4. Trapezoid ligament
5. Conoid ligament
6. Glenoid labrum

1. **Supraspinatus**
   O: Supraspinatus fossa of scapula.
   I: Greater tuberosity of humerus.
   A: Initiates abduction of humerus (raising arm to side), stabilizes head of humerus in socket of shoulder joint.

2. **Subscapularis**
   O: Front surface of scapula in subscapular fossa.
   I: Lesser tuberosity of humerus.
   A: Internally rotates humerus, stabilizes head of humerus in socket of shoulder joint.

3. **Teres minor**
   O: Upper part of lateral border of scapula.
   I: Back and lower part of greater tuberosity of humerus.
   A: Externally rotates humerus, stabilizes head of humerus in socket of shoulder joint.

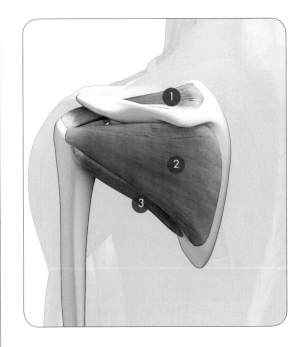

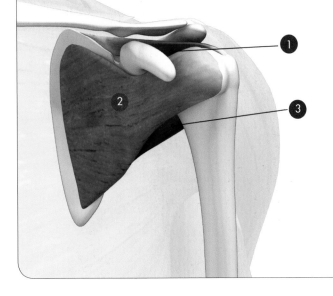

1. **Supraspinatus**
   O: Supraspinatus fossa of scapula.
   I: Greater tuberosity of humerus.
   A: Initiates abduction of humerus (raising arm to side), stabilizes head of humerus in socket of shoulder joint.

2. **Infraspinatus**
   O: Infraspinatus fossa of scapula.
   I: Greater tuberosity of humerus.
   A: Externally rotates shoulder.

3. **Teres minor**
   O: Upper part of lateral border of scapula.
   I: Back and lower part of greater tuberosity of humerus.
   A: Externally rotates humerus, stabilizes head of humerus in socket of shoulder joint.

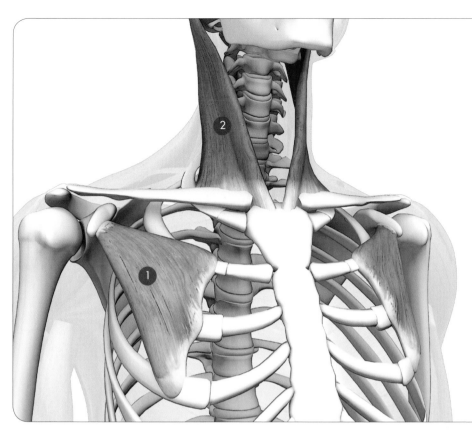

1 **Pectoralis minor**

O: Front of ribs 3-5.

I: Coracoid process of scapula.

A: Rolls shoulder forward and down (via scapula), lifts ribcage when scapula is stabilized by rhomboids (expands chest) through closed chain contraction.

2 **Sternocleidomastoid**

O: Sternal head: manubrium of sternum; clavicular head: upper surface of medial third of clavicle.

I: Mastoid process behind and below ear.

A: When both sides contract together flexes neck and tilts head forward; if head is stabilized, lifts upper ribcage during inhalation; contracting one side tilts head to side of muscle, rotates head to face away from muscle.

1 **Pectoralis major**

O: Sternocostal head: front of manubrium and body of sternum; clavicular head: medial half of clavicle.

I: Outer edge of bicipital groove on upper humerus.

A: Adducts and internally rotates humerus. Sternocostal head draws humerus down and across the body towards opposite hip. Clavicular head forward flexes and internally rotates the humerus, draws humerus across body towards opposite shoulder.

2 **Coracobrachialis**

O: Coracoid process of scapula.

I: Inner surface of humerus at mid-shaft.

A: Assists pectoralis in adduction of humerus and shoulder.

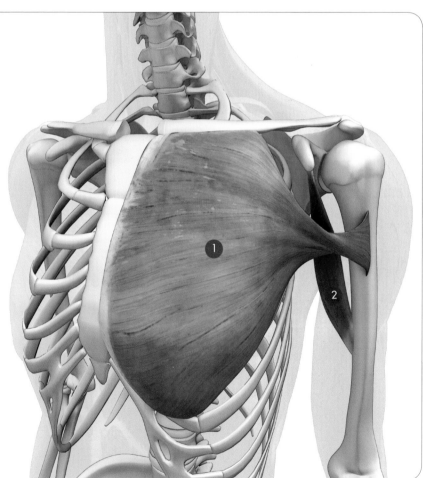

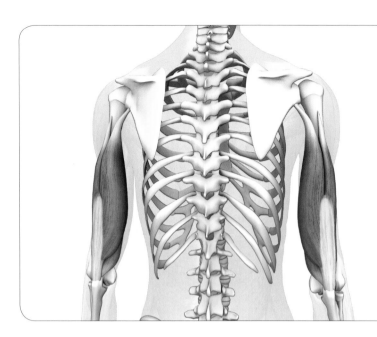

Triceps brachii

O: Long head from infraglenoid tubercle at bottom of shoulder socket; medial and lateral heads from posterior surface of humerus and intermuscular septum.

I: Olecranon process of ulna.

A: Extends elbow, long head moves arm back and adducts it.

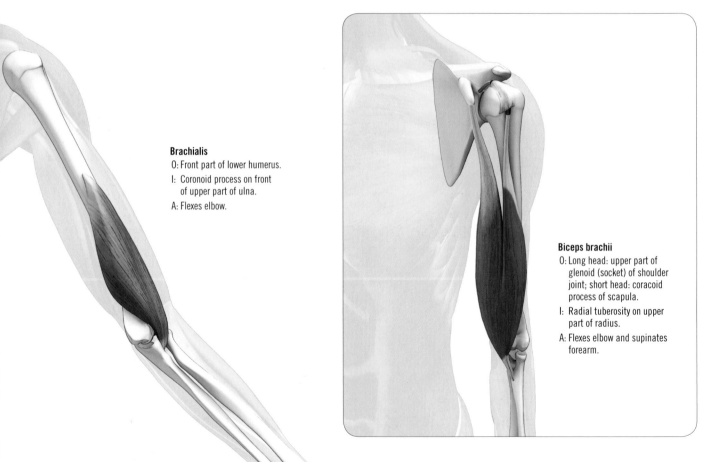

Brachialis

O: Front part of lower humerus.

I: Coronoid process on front of upper part of ulna.

A: Flexes elbow.

Biceps brachii

O: Long head: upper part of glenoid (socket) of shoulder joint; short head: coracoid process of scapula.

I: Radial tuberosity on upper part of radius.

A: Flexes elbow and supinates forearm.

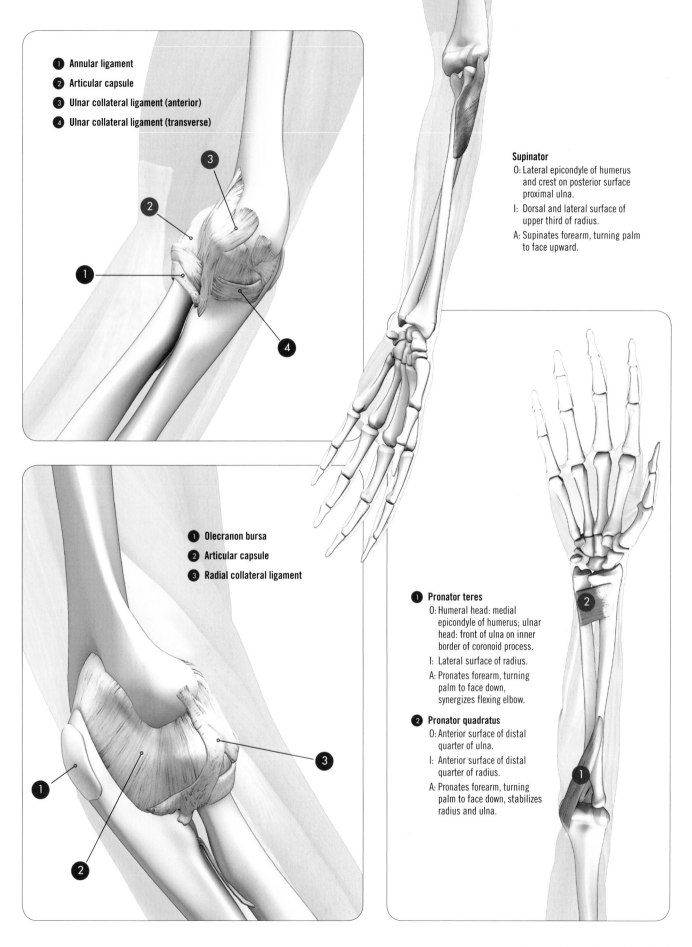

1 Annular ligament
2 Articular capsule
3 Ulnar collateral ligament (anterior)
4 Ulnar collateral ligament (transverse)

1 Olecranon bursa
2 Articular capsule
3 Radial collateral ligament

Supinator

O: Lateral epicondyle of humerus and crest on posterior surface proximal ulna.

I: Dorsal and lateral surface of upper third of radius.

A: Supinates forearm, turning palm to face upward.

1 Pronator teres

O: Humeral head: medial epicondyle of humerus; ulnar head: front of ulna on inner border of coronoid process.

I: Lateral surface of radius.

A: Pronates forearm, turning palm to face down, synergizes flexing elbow.

2 Pronator quadratus

O: Anterior surface of distal quarter of ulna.

I: Anterior surface of distal quarter of radius.

A: Pronates forearm, turning palm to face down, stabilizes radius and ulna.

❶ Flexor digitorum profundis

O: Upper two thirds of anterior and medial surface of ulna and interosseous membrane (between radius and ulna).

I: Palmar (anterior) surface of distal phalanges of fingers.

A: Flexes distal phalanges, synergizes flexion of more proximal phalanges and wrist.

❷ Flexor pollicis longus

O: Anterior surface of mid-shaft of radius, coronoid process of ulna, medial epicondyle.

I: Palmar (anterior) surface of distal phalanx of thumb.

A: Flexes thumb and synergizes flexion of wrist.

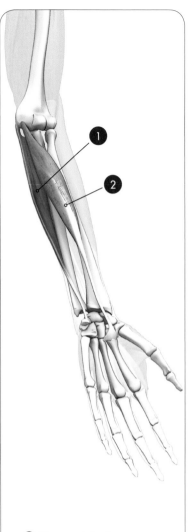

Flexor digitorum superficialis

O: Medial epicondyle, coronoid process of ulna, upper anterior border of radius.

I: Two slips of tendon insert onto either side of middle phalanges of four fingers.

A: Flexes middle phalanges of fingers, synergizes wrist flexion.

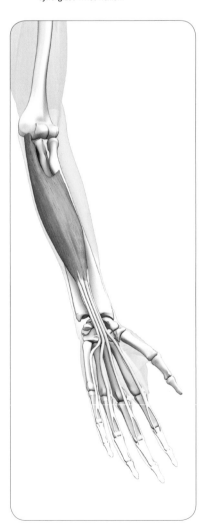

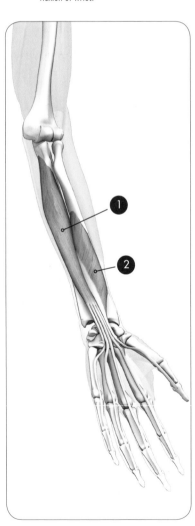

❶ Flexor carpi ulnaris

O: Medial epicondyle of humerus, medial border and upper two thirds of ulna.

I: Pisiform bone of wrist, base of fifth metacarpal.

A: Flexes and adducts wrist, synergizes elbow flexion.

❷ Flexor carpi radialis

O: Medial epicondyle of humerus.

I: Base of second metacarpal.

A: Flexes and abducts wrist, synergizes elbow flexion and pronation.

1. Brachioradialis
O: Lateral supracondylar ridge of humerus.

I: Lower outside surface of radius, proximal to styloid process.

A: Flexes elbow.

2. Extensor carpi radialis longus
O: Lateral supracondylar ridge of humerus.

I: Dorsal surface of base of second metacarpal.

A: Extends and abducts wrist.

3. Extensor carpi radialis brevis
O: Lateral epicondyle via common extensor tendon.

I: Dorsal surface of base of third metacarpal.

A: Extends and abducts wrist.

4. Extensor carpi ulnaris
O: Lateral epicondyle via common extensor tendon.

I: Base of fifth metacarpal.

A: Extends and adducts wrist.

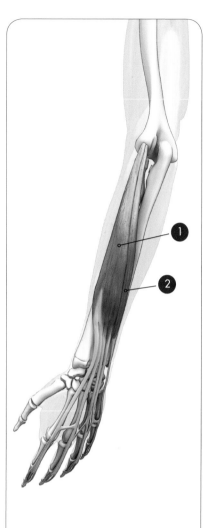

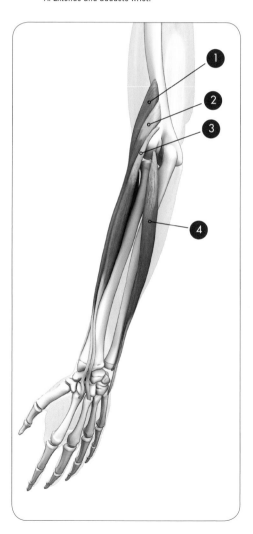

1. Extensor digitorum
O: Lateral epicondyle via common extensor tendon.

I: Dorsal surfaces of phalanges of all four fingers.

A: Extends fingers, synergizes finger abduction away from midline.

2. Extensor digiti minimi
O: Lateral epicondyle via common extensor tendon.

I: Combines with tendon of extensor digitorum to insert onto dorsum of little finger.

A: Extends little finger.

1. Abductor pollicis longus
O: Posterior surface of ulna and radius covering middle third of bones, interosseous membrane.

I: Lateral surface of first metacarpal.

A: Extends and abducts thumb, synergist of forearm supination and wrist flexion.

2. Extensor pollicis brevis
O: Posterior surface of distal radius, interosseous membrane.

I: Dorsal surface of base of proximal phalanx of thumb.

A: Extends thumb, synergizes wrist abduction.

3. Extensor pollicis longus
O: Posterior surface of middle third of ulna, interosseous membrane.

I: Dorsal surface at base of distal phalanx of thumb.

A: Extends thumb, synergizes wrist extension.

4. Extensor indicis
O: Posterior surface of distal ulna, interosseous membrane.

I: Dorsal aponeurosis of index finger, onto proximal phalanx.

A: Extends index finger.

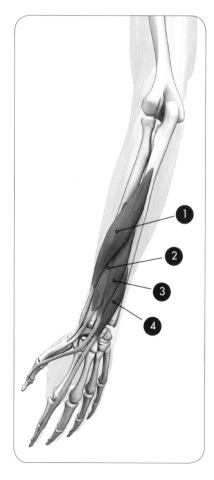

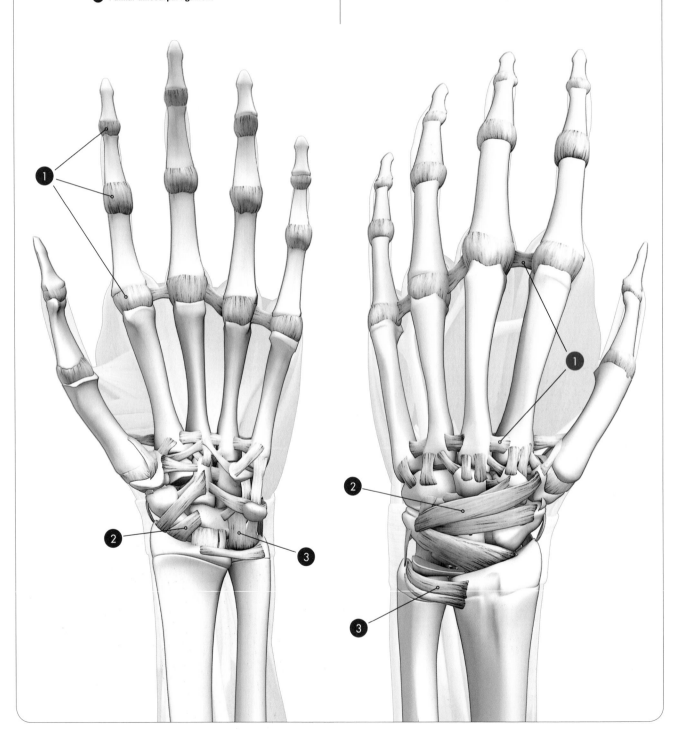

1 Metacarpophalangeal and
interphalangeal joint capsules

2 Palmar radiocarpal and intercarpal ligaments

3 Palmar ulnocarpal ligament

1 Transverse metacarpal ligaments

2 Dorsal intercarpal ligaments

3 Dorsal radioulnar ligament

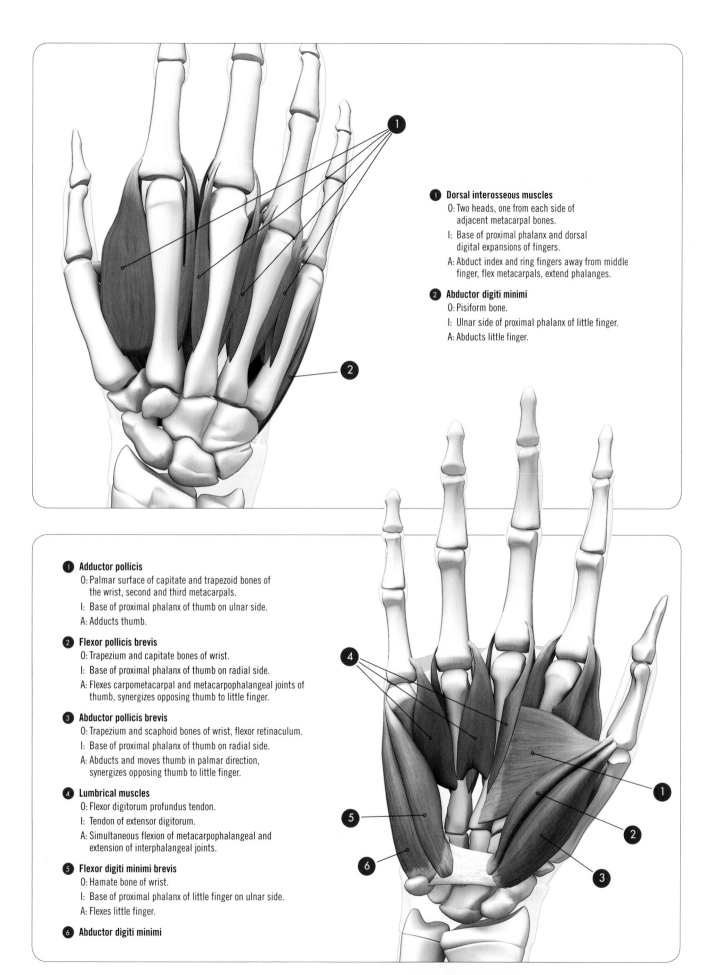

1 Dorsal interosseous muscles

O: Two heads, one from each side of adjacent metacarpal bones.

I: Base of proximal phalanx and dorsal digital expansions of fingers.

A: Abduct index and ring fingers away from middle finger, flex metacarpals, extend phalanges.

2 Abductor digiti minimi

O: Pisiform bone.

I: Ulnar side of proximal phalanx of little finger.

A: Abducts little finger.

1 Adductor pollicis

O: Palmar surface of capitate and trapezoid bones of the wrist, second and third metacarpals.

I: Base of proximal phalanx of thumb on ulnar side.

A: Adducts thumb.

2 Flexor pollicis brevis

O: Trapezium and capitate bones of wrist.

I: Base of proximal phalanx of thumb on radial side.

A: Flexes carpometacarpal and metacarpophalangeal joints of thumb, synergizes opposing thumb to little finger.

3 Abductor pollicis brevis

O: Trapezium and scaphoid bones of wrist, flexor retinaculum.

I: Base of proximal phalanx of thumb on radial side.

A: Abducts and moves thumb in palmar direction, synergizes opposing thumb to little finger.

4 Lumbrical muscles

O: Flexor digitorum profundus tendon.

I: Tendon of extensor digitorum.

A: Simultaneous flexion of metacarpophalangeal and extension of interphalangeal joints.

5 Flexor digiti minimi brevis

O: Hamate bone of wrist.

I: Base of proximal phalanx of little finger on ulnar side.

A: Flexes little finger.

6 Abductor digiti minimi

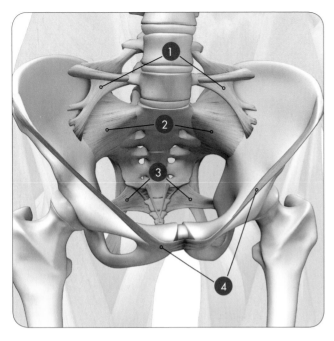

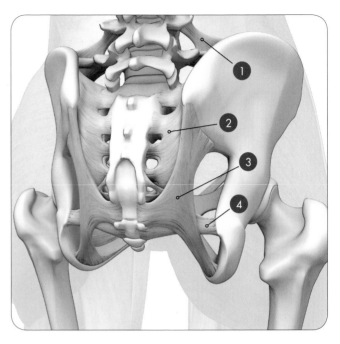

1 Iliolumbar ligament   **3** Sacrospinous ligament

2 Sacroiliac ligament   **4** Inguinal ligament

1 Iliolumbar ligament   **3** Sacrotuberous ligament

2 Sacroiliac ligament   **4** Sacrospinous ligament

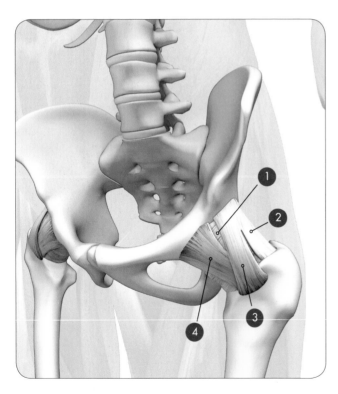

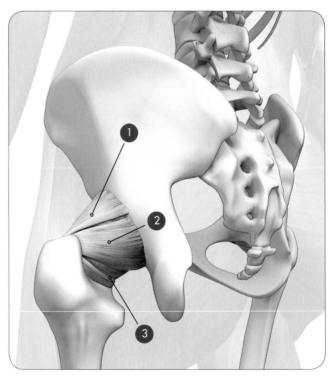

1 Zona orbicularis (hip capsule)   **3** Anterior iliofemoral ligament

2 Lateral iliofemoral ligament   **4** Pubofemoral ligament

1 Lateral iliofemoral ligament   **3** Zona orbicularis (hip capsule)

2 Ischiofemoral ligament

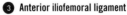

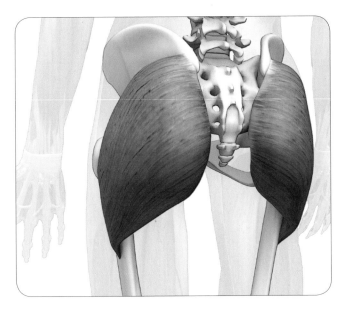

Gluteus maximus

O: Posterolateral surface of ilium and lateral surface of the sacrum.

I: Upper fibers onto iliotibial tract; lower fibers onto gluteal tuberosity.

A: Extends, externally rotates, and stabilizes hip.

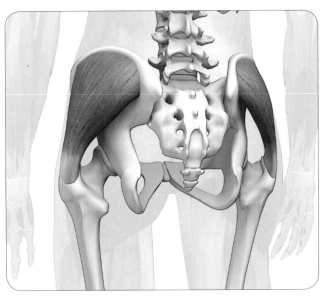

Gluteus medius

O: Outer surface of ilium.

I: Greater trochanter.

A: Abducts hip, anterior fibers internally rotate and flex hip, posterior fibers externally rotate and extend hip.

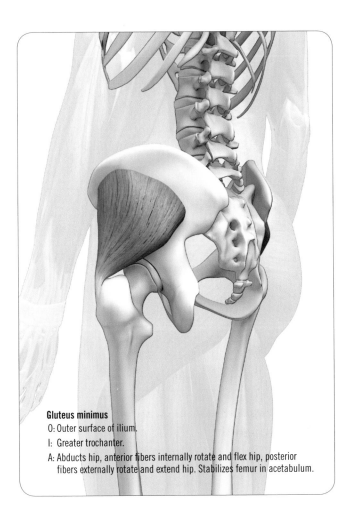

Gluteus minimus

O: Outer surface of ilium.

I: Greater trochanter.

A: Abducts hip, anterior fibers internally rotate and flex hip, posterior fibers externally rotate and extend hip. Stabilizes femur in acetabulum.

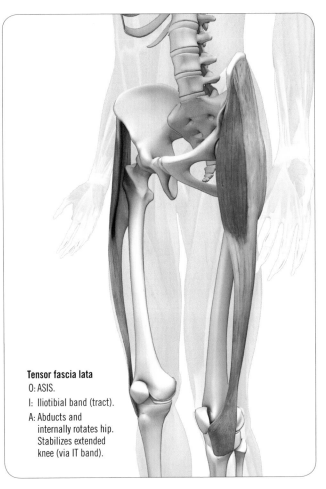

Tensor fascia lata

O: ASIS.

I: Iliotibial band (tract).

A: Abducts and internally rotates hip. Stabilizes extended knee (via IT band).

1 Piriformis
O: Posterior surface of sacrum.
I: Greater trochanter.
A: Externally rotates, abducts, extends, and stabilizes hip.

2 Superior gemellus
O: Ischial spine.
I: Greater trochanter.
A: Externally rotates and adducts hip.

3 Obturator internus
O: Obturator membrane and ischium.
I: Greater trochanter.
A: Externally rotates and adducts hip.

4 Inferior gemellus
O: Ischial tuberosity.
I: Greater trochanter.
A: Externally rotates and adducts hip.

5 Quadratus femoris
O: Ischial tuberosity.
I: Intertrochanteric crest.
A: Externally rotates and adducts hip.

6 Obturator externus
O: Obturator membrane and ischium.
I: Greater trochanter.
A: Externally rotates and adducts hip.

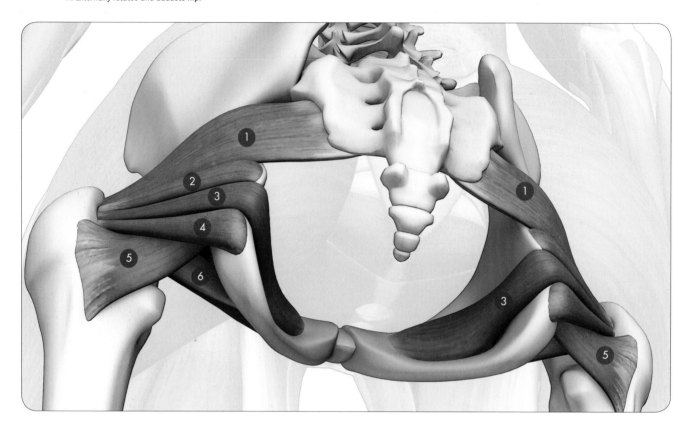

1 Psoas major
O: T12-L4 vertebral bodies and discs.
I: Lesser trochanter.
A: Flexes and externally rotates hip, stabilizes lumbar spine.

2 Iliacus
O: Inner surface of ilium.
I: Lesser trochanter.
A: Flexes and externally rotates hip, with psoas major tilts pelvis forward.

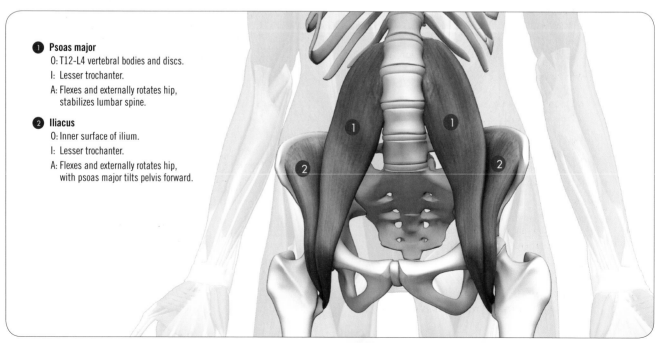

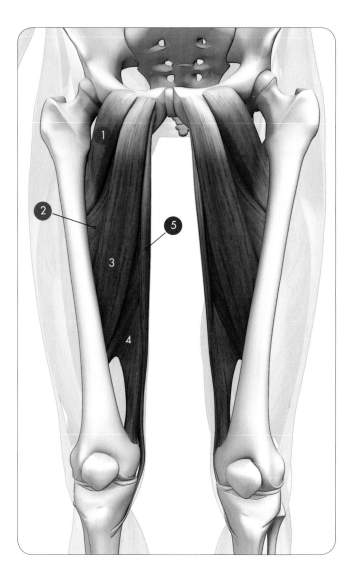

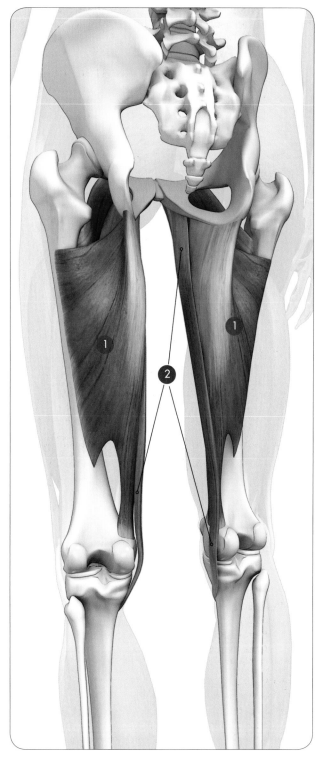

1 **Pectineus**

O: Pubic bone.

I: Linea aspera of femur.

A: Adducts, externally rotates, and synergizes femur flexion.

2 **Adductor brevis**

O: Pubic bone.

I: Linea aspera of femur.

A: Adducts and flexes femur, stabilizes pelvis.

3 **Adductor longus**

O: Pubic bone.

I: Linea aspera of femur.

A: Adducts and flexes femur, stabilizes pelvis.

4 **Adductor magnus**

O: Pubic bone and ischial tuberosity.

I: Linea aspera and medial epicondyle of femur.

A: Adducts, externally rotates, and extends femur.

5 **Gracilis**

O: Pubic bone.

I: Medial tibia.

A: Adducts and flexes hip, flexes and internally rotates knee.

1 Adductor magnus

2 Gracilis

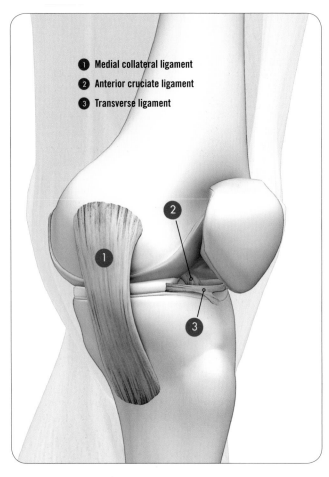

1 Medial collateral ligament
2 Anterior cruciate ligament
3 Transverse ligament

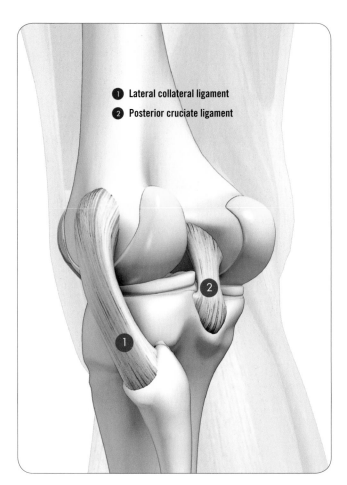

1 Lateral collateral ligament
2 Posterior cruciate ligament

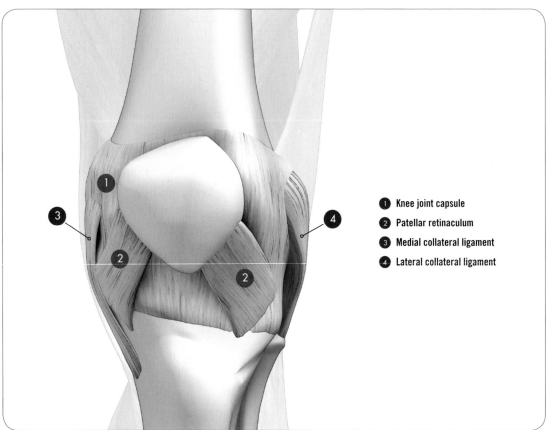

1 Knee joint capsule
2 Patellar retinaculum
3 Medial collateral ligament
4 Lateral collateral ligament

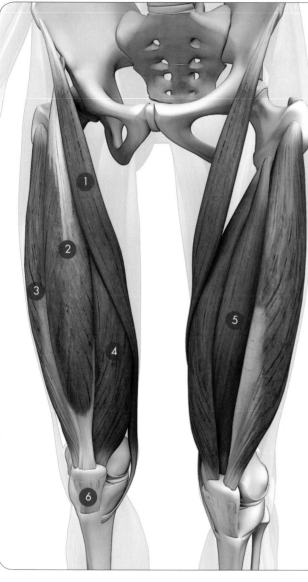

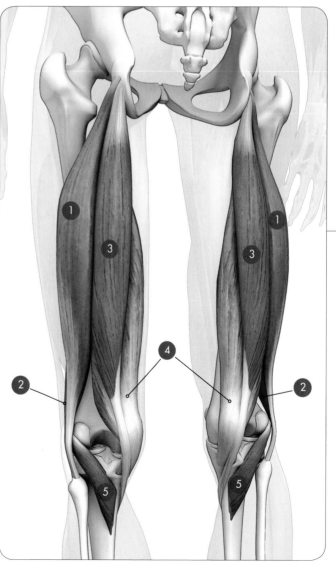

1. **Sartorius**

   O: ASIS.

   I: Pes anserinus of medial tibia.

   A: Flexes, abducts, and externally rotates hip; flexes and internally rotates knee.

2. **Rectus femoris**

   O: ASIS.

   I: Anterior tibia via patellar tendon.

   A: Flexes hip, tilts pelvis forward, extends knee.

3. **Vastus lateralis**

   O: Lateral femur.

   I: Anterior tibia via patellar tendon.

   A: Extends knee.

4. **Vastus medialis**

   O: Medial femur.

   I: Anterior tibia via patellar tendon.

   A: Extends knee.

5. **Vastus intermedius**

   O: Anterior femur.

   I: Anterior tibia via patellar tendon.

   A: Extends knee.

6. **Patellar tendon**

1. **Biceps femoris long head**

   O: Ischial tuberosity.

   I: Fibular head.

   A: Extends hip, flexes and externally rotates knee.

2. **Biceps femoris short head**

   O: Posterior surface of femur.

   I: Fibular head.

   A: Extends hip, flexes and externally rotates knee.

3. **Semitendinosus**

   O: Ischial tuberosity.

   I: Pes anserinus of medial tibia.

   A: Extends hip, flexes and internally rotates knee.

4. **Semimembranosus**

   O: Ischial tuberosity.

   I: Back of medial tibial condyle.

   A: Extends hip, flexes and internally rotates knee.

5. **Popliteus**

   O: Lateral femoral condyle.

   I: Posterior surface of tibia, below knee joint.

   A: Flexes and internally rotates knee.

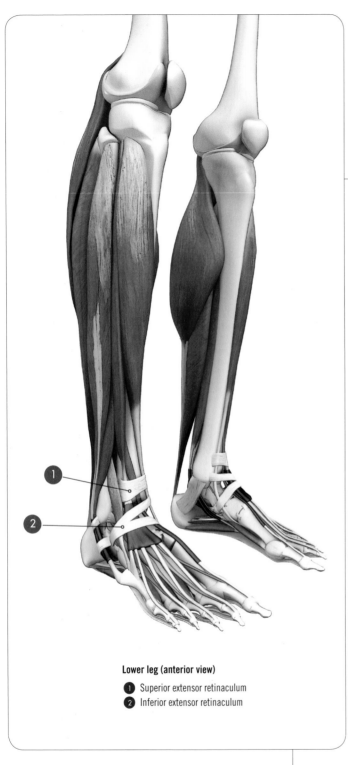

Lower leg (anterior view)

1 Superior extensor retinaculum
2 Inferior extensor retinaculum

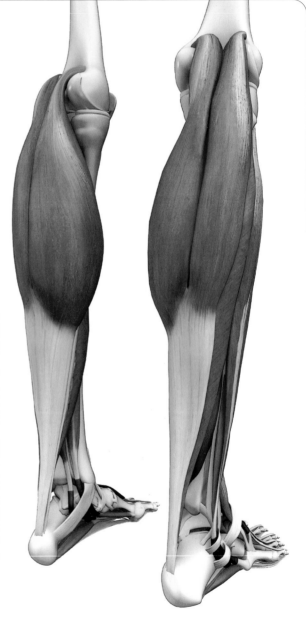

Lower leg (posterior view)

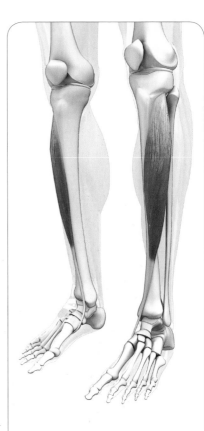

1 Peroneus longus

O: Head and proximal two thirds of lateral fibula.

I: Base of first metacarpal and medial cuneiform.

A: Plantar flexes ankle and everts subtalar joint, supports transverse arch of foot.

2 Peroneus brevis

O: Distal half of lateral surface of fibula, intermuscular membrane.

I: Base of fifth metatarsal.

A: Plantar flexes ankle and everts subtalar joint.

3 Peroneus tertius

O: Front of distal fibula.

I: Base of fifth metatarsal.

A: Dorsiflexes ankle and everts subtalar joint.

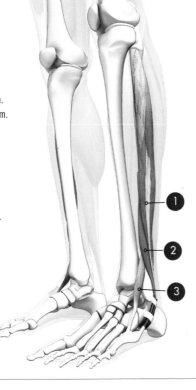

Tibialis anterior

O: Upper two thirds of anterior tibia and interosseous membrane.

I: Medial cuneiform, base of first metatarsal.

A: Dorsiflexes ankle, inverts subtalar joint.

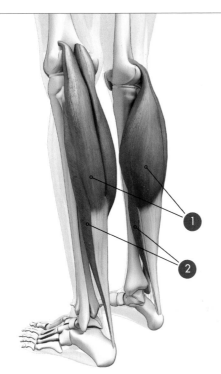

1 Gastrocnemius

O: Medial head from medial epicondyle of femur; lateral head from lateral epicondyle.

I: Calcaneous via Achilles tendon.

A: Plantar flexes and inverts ankle, flexes knee.

2 Soleus

O: Posterior surface of head and neck of fibula.

I: Calcaneous via Achilles tendon.

A: Plantar flexes ankle, inverts subtalar joint, and flexes knee.

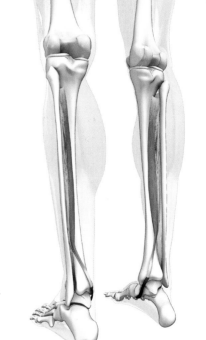

Tibialis posterior

O: Interosseous membrane between tibia and fibula.

I: Navicular, cuneiform bones, and second through fourth metatarsals.

A: Plantar flexes ankle, inverts subtalar joint, and supports longitudinal and transverse foot arches.

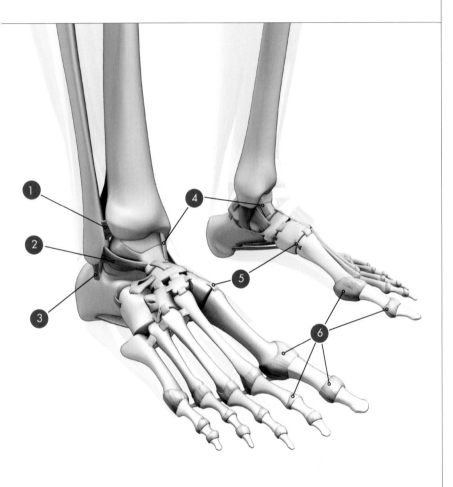

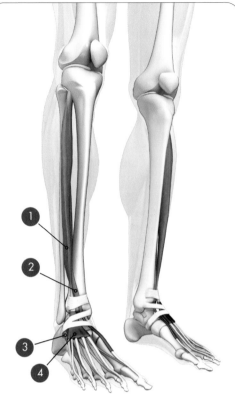

1 Anterior tibiofibular ligament   4 Anterior tibiotalar ligament

2 Anterior talofibular ligament   5 Dorsal metatarsal ligaments

3 Calcaneofibular ligament   6 Interphalangeal joint capsules

1 **Extensor digitorum longus**
   O: Lateral tibial condyle, fibular head, interosseous membrane.
   I: Dorsal aponeurosis and bases of the distal phalanges of second through fifth toes.
   A: Dorsiflexes ankle, everts subtalar joint, and extends metatarsophalangeal and interphalangeal joints of toes.

2 **Extensor hallucis longus**
   O: Medial surface of fibula, interosseous membrane.
   I: Dorsal aponeurosis and base of distal phalanx of big toe.
   A: Dorsiflexes ankle, everts subtalar joint, and extends big toe.

3 **Extensor digitorum brevis**
   O: Dorsal surface of calcaneous.
   I: Dorsal aponeurosis and bases of middle phalanges of second through fourth toes.
   A: Extends metatarsophalangeal and proximal interphalangeal joints of second through fourth toes.

4 **Extensor tendons sheath**

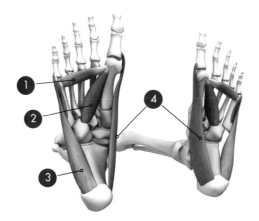

1 **Adductor hallucis (transverse head)**

O: Metatarsophalangeal joints of third through fifth toes.

I: Base of proximal phalanx of big toe via sesamoid.

A: Adducts and flexes big toe, supports transverse foot arch.

2 **Adductor hallucis (oblique head)**

O: Bases of second through fourth metatarsals, lateral cuneiform, and cuboid.

I: Base of proximal phalanx of big toe via sesamoid.

A: Adducts and flexes big toe, supports longitudinal foot arch.

3 **Abductor digiti minimi**

O: Calcaneous, plantar aponeurosis.

I: Base of proximal phalanx of little toe.

A: Flexes metatarsophalangeal joint and abducts little toe, supports longitudinal foot arch.

4 **Abductor hallucis**

O: Calcaneous, plantar aponeurosis.

I: Base of proximal phalanx of big toe.

A: Flexes and abducts big toe, supports longitudinal foot arch.

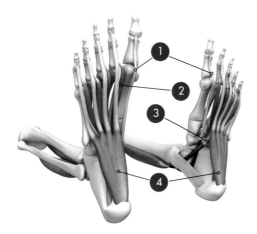

1 **Flexor hallucis longus**

O: Posterior surface of fibula, interosseous membrane.

I: Base of distal phalanx of big toe.

A: Plantar flexes ankle, inverts subtalar joint, flexes big toe, supports longitudinal foot arch.

2 **Lumbrical muscles**

O: Medial borders of flexor digitorum longus tendons.

I: Dorsal aponeurosis of second through fifth toes.

A: Flexes metatarsophalangeal and extends interphalangeal joints of second through fifth toes, adducts toe.

3 **Flexor digitorum longus**

O: Posterior surface of tibia.

I: Bases of distal phalanges of second through fifth toes.

A: Plantar flexes ankle, inverts subtalar joint, plantar flexes toes.

4 **Flexor digitorum brevis**

O: Calcaneous, plantar aponeurosis.

I: Middle phalanges of second through fifth toes.

A: Flexes toes, supports longitudinal foot arch.

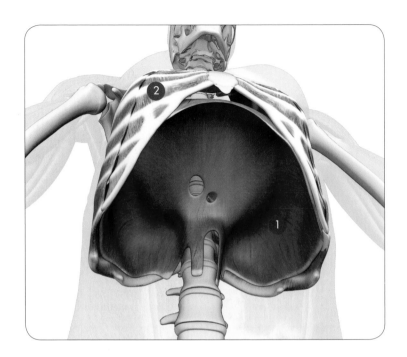

1 **Diaphragm**

O: Lower margin of costal arch, posterior surface of xiphoid process of sternum, arcuate ligament of aorta, L1-3 vertebral bodies.

I: Central tendon.

A: Primary muscle of respiration, aids in compressing abdomen.

2 **Intercostals**

O: Internal intercostals from surface of upper margin of rib; external intercostals from lower margin of rib.

I: Internals insert on lower margin of next higher rib; externals insert on upper margin of next lower rib.

A: Internal intercostals lower ribs during exhalation; externals raise ribs during inhalation.

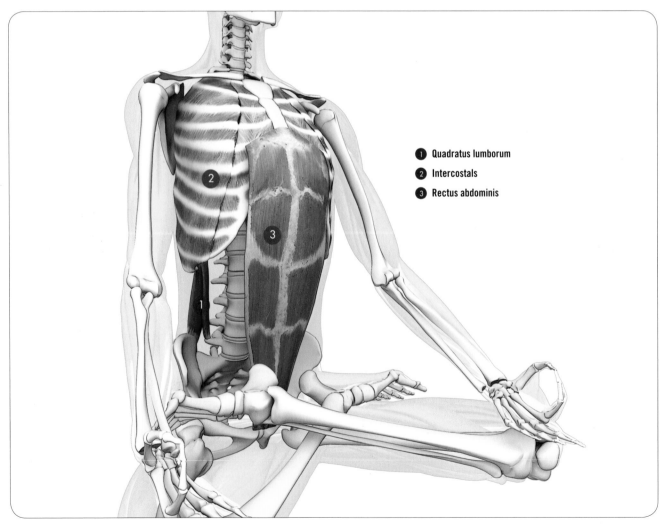

1 Quadratus lumborum

2 Intercostals

3 Rectus abdominis

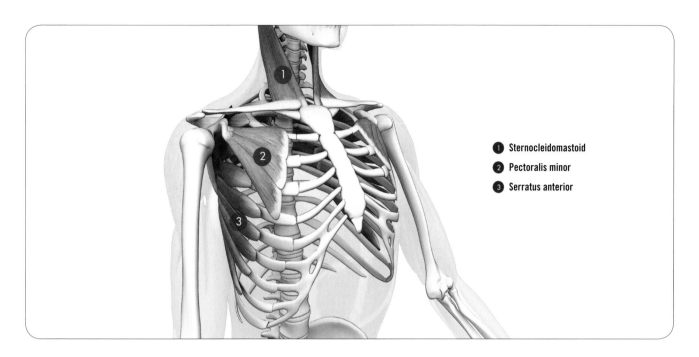

1 Sternocleidomastoid

2 Pectoralis minor

3 Serratus anterior

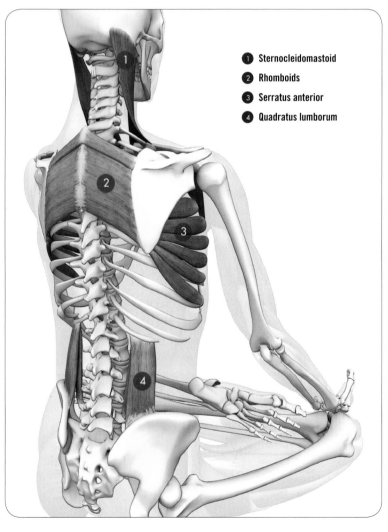

1 Sternocleidomastoid

2 Rhomboids

3 Serratus anterior

4 Quadratus lumborum

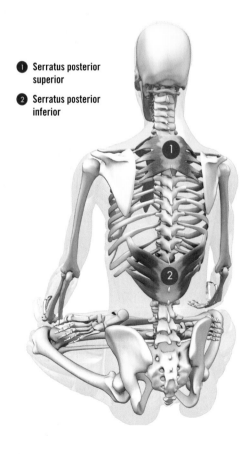

1 Serratus posterior superior

2 Serratus posterior inferior

INDEX OF MUSCLES AND LIGAMENTS

GLOSSARY OF TERMS

Abduction Moving away from the midline.

Accessory muscles of breathing Muscles that attach to the ribcage and thorax that can be used to augment the action of the diaphragm for inhalation and exhalation. These include the rhomboids, pectorals, quadratus lumborum, sternocleidomastoid, and intercostals (among others).

Active insufficiency A condition in which a muscle is shortened or lengthened to a point where it can no longer effectively move a joint. For example, in Kurmasana the hips are fully flexed and so the psoas muscle is shortened to a point where it cannot effectively flex the hips further. At such times, other parts of the body must be used for leverage, such as the arms under the knees.

Adduction Moving toward the midline.

Agonist The muscle that contracts to produce a certain action about a joint (sometimes referred to as the prime mover). For example, the brachialis contracts to flex the elbow joint.

Alveoli Sac-like spherical structures with thin membrane-like walls through which gas exchange occurs in the lungs.

Anatomy The study of the structure of living things. Musculoskeletal anatomy studies the bones, ligaments, muscles, and tendons.

Antagonist The muscle that opposes the action of the agonist muscle and produces the opposite action about a joint. For example, the hamstrings are the antagonists to the quadriceps for extending the knee.

Anteversion Tilting forward.

Aponeurosis A fibrous thickening of fascia that forms the attachment for muscles. For example, the abdominal muscles attach to the linea alba, an aponeurotic thickening at the front of the abdomen.

Appendicular skeleton Composed of the shoulder (pectoral girdle) and upper extremities and pelvis and lower extremities.

Asana Sanskrit term for body position in yoga (yogasana).

Autonomic nervous system Part of the nervous system that functions largely unconsciously to control breathing, heart rate, blood pressure, digestion, perspiration, and other functions. It is divided into the sympathetic (fight or flight) and parasympathetic (rest and digest) nervous systems.

Axial skeleton Composed of the skull, spine, and ribcage.

Bandha Sanskrit term referring to binding, locking, or stabilizing. Co-activating muscle groups can be used to form bandhas in yoga postures.

Biomechanics The application of mechanical physics to the body. For example, contracting the biceps flexes the elbow joint.

Carpals The bones of the wrist, including the scaphoid, lunate, triquetrum, hamate, capitate, trapezoid, and trapezium.

Center of gravity The center of an object's weight distribution and at which point an object is in balance.

Center of gravity projection An extension of the force of gravity downward and away from the body. For example, in Warrior III the center of gravity is projected out through the arms and the back leg, balancing the pose.

Chakra Wheel-like centers or concentrations of energy within the subtle body. They may correspond to collections of nerves such as the lumbosacral plexus (for the first and second chakras).

Closed chain contraction/movement The origin of the muscle moves and the insertion remains stationary. For example, the psoas contracts to flex the trunk in Trikonasana.

Co-contraction/co-activation Simultaneously contracting agonist and antagonist muscles to stabilize a joint. For example, co-activating the peroneus longus and brevis and the tibialis posterior muscles stabilizes the ankle joint.

Core muscles Composed of the transversus abdominis, internal and external obliques, rectus abdominis, erector spinae, psoas, gluteus maximus, and pelvic diaphragm.

Drishti Sanskrit term for focus of vision or gaze.

Eccentric contraction The muscle generates tension (contracts) while lengthening.

Erector spinae The group of three deep back muscles that run parallel to the spinal column, including the spinalis, longissimus, and iliocostalis muscles.

Eversion Rotating the sole of the foot (via the ankle) away from the midline of the body. This is associated with pronation (internal rotation) of the forefoot.

Extension Joint movement that increases space and distance between skeletal segments, bringing them farther apart.

Facilitated stretching A powerful method of stretching in which the muscle is first taken out to its full length and then contracted for several moments. This stimulates the Golgi tendon organ and produces the "relaxation response," causing the muscle to relax and lengthen. It is also known as PNF.

Fascia Connective tissue that surrounds, separates, and binds muscles to each other. This can also form an aponeurosis for muscle attachment.

Flexion Joint movement that decreases space between skeletal segments and draws them closer together.

Floating ribs Five pairs of ribs that articulate posteriorly with the vertebrae and attach to the costal cartilage anteriorly.

Forefoot The region of the foot distal to the midfoot. It is composed of the metatarsal and phalangeal bones (and their corresponding joints). Motion includes toe flexion and extension and deepening of the foot arches.

Glenohumeral joint Ball and socket synovial joint where the head (ball) of the humerus articulates with the glenoid fossa (socket) of the scapula.

Golgi tendon organ A sensory receptor located at the muscle-tendon junction that detects changes in tension. This information is conveyed to the central nervous system, which then signals the muscle to relax, providing "slack" in the muscle. This protects against the tendon being torn from the bone. The Golgi tendon organ is central to PNF or facilitated stretching.

Hindfoot Typically refers to the calcaneous and talus bones. The joint for the hindfoot is the subtalar joint, which is responsible for everting and inverting the foot. For example, the hindfoot is inverted in the back leg in Warrior I.

Iliotibial tract Fibrous fascial structure that runs on the outside of the thigh and blends into the lateral portion of the knee capsule. This forms the attachment for the tensor fascia lata and part of the gluteus maximus muscles.

Impingement Narrowing or encroachment of the space between two bones. It can cause inflammation and pain. For example, a nerve root can become impinged by a herniated intervertebral disc. You can also have impingement between the humeral head and the acromion, causing pain in the shoulder.

Insertion The distal site where a muscle attaches to a bone (via a tendon), usually farther from the midline of the body and more mobile than the muscle origin at its opposite end.

Inversion Rotating the sole of the foot towards the midline of the body (turning it inward). This is associated with supination (external rotation) of the forefoot.

Isometric contraction The muscle generates tension but does not shorten, and the bones do not move.

Isotonic contraction The muscle shortens while maintaining constant tension through a range of motion.

Kriya Sanskrit term for action or activity.

Leverage Creating a mechanical advantage based on the length of the lever. For example, placing the hand on the outside of the foot in Parivrtta Trikonasana uses the length of the arm for leverage to turn the body.

Line of action A line through which forces act or are directed within the body. For example, there is a line of action extending from the tips of the fingers to the heel in Utthita Parsvakonasana.

Metacarpals The intermediate region of the hand between the carpus (wrist) and the fingers, i.e., the five bones of the palms of the hands.

Midfoot The intermediate region of the foot between the hindfoot and forefoot. It is composed of the navicular, the cuboid, and three cuneiform bones. Motion includes contribution to supination and pronation of the forefoot.

Mudra Sanskrit term for seal; similar to a bandha. It is often performed with the hands by bringing the fingertips together in a specific way. Other mudras are created by combining bandhas throughout the body.

Muscle spindle A sensory receptor within the muscle belly that detects changes in length and tension in the muscle. This information is conveyed to the central nervous system which can then signal the muscle to contract to resist stretching. This reflex protects against tearing the muscle.

Open chain contraction/movement The insertion of the muscle moves and the origin remains stationary. For example, the deltoids contract to lift the arms in Warrior II.

Origin The proximal site where a muscle attaches to a bone (via a tendon), usually closer to the midline of the body and less mobile than the muscle insertion on the bone at its opposite end.

Parivrtta Revolving, twisted, or turning version of a pose. For example, Parivrtta Trikonasana is the revolving version of Trikonasana (Triangle Pose).

Pelvic girdle The ilium, ischium, pubic bones, and pubic symphysis.

Physiology The study of the functional processes of living things. Most physiological processes take place unconsciously but can be influenced by the conscious mind. Examples include breathing and facilitated stretching.

PNF Proprioceptive neuromuscular facilitation. Also known as *facilitated stretching*. (See facilitated stretching.)

Posterior kinetic chain Composed of a group of interconnecting ligaments, tendons, and muscles on the back of the body. Includes the hamstrings, gluteus maximus, erector spinae, trapezius, latissimus, and posterior deltoids.

Pranayama Yogic art of controlling the breath.

Prime mover The muscle that contracts to directly produce a desired movement. For example, the quadriceps contracts to extend the knee joint. The term is sometimes used interchangeably with 'agonist muscle.'

Radial deviation Tilting the hand toward the index-finger side or away from the midline of the body.

Reciprocal inhibition A phenomenon whereby the brain signals an agonist muscle to contract, and a simultaneous inhibitory signal is sent to the antagonist muscle, causing it to relax. This physiological process takes place unconsciously.

Retroversion Tilting backward.

Rotation Joint movement around a longitudinal axis. For example, we externally rotate the humerus bones (longitudinal axis) to turn the palms to face up in Savasana.

Scapulohumeral rhythm Simultaneous movements at the glenohumeral and scapulothoracic joints that function together to abduct and flex the shoulders. For example, scapulohumeral rhythm takes place when we raise the arms overhead in Urdhva Hastasana.

Shoulder girdle The clavicles and scapulae.

Synergist A muscle that assists and fine-tunes the action of the agonist or prime mover. It can be used to produce the same action, although generally not as efficiently. For example, the pectineus muscle synergizes the psoas in flexing the hip joint.

True ribs Seven pairs of ribs that articulate posteriorly with the vertebrae and anteriorly with the sternum.

Ulnar deviation Tilting the hand toward the little-finger side or midline of the body.

SANSKRIT PRONUNCIATION AND POSE INDEX

Sanskrit	Pronunciation	Pages
Ardha Badha Padma Paschimottanasana	[ARE-dah BAH-dah pod-MAH POSH-ee-moh-tun-AWS-ah-nah]	16, **144**
Ardha Matsyendrasana	[ARE-dah MOT-see-en-DRAHS-anna]	98
Ardha Padmasana	[ARE-dah pod-MAHS-anna]	98
Baddha Konasana	[BAH-dah cone-NAHS-anna]	28, **33**, 40
Dandasana	[don-DAHS-anna]	34, 39, 42, 98, **106**
Hanumanasana	[hah-new-mahn-AHS-anna]	**89**, 14
Janu Sirsasana	[JAH-new shear-SHAHS-anna]	19, **114**, 122, 135, 144, 146
Krounchasana	[crown-CHAHS-anna]	7, 9, **136**
Kurmasana	[koohr-MAH-sah-nah]	6, **74**
Marichyasana III	[mar-ee-chee-AHS-anna]	68
Navasana	[nuh-VAHS-anna]	**153**, 160
Padmasana	[pod-MAHS-anna]	16, 33, **96**, 144, 146, 151
Parighasana	[par-ee-GOSS-anna]	**80**
Parighasana I	[par-ee-GOSS-anna]	82
Parivrtta Trikonasana	[par-ee-vrit-tah trik-cone-AHS-anna]	66
Paschimottanasana	[POSH-ee-moh-tan-AHS-anna]	7, 10, 13, 40, 108, **122**
Sukhasana	[SOOK-ahs-anna]	**26**, 96
Supta Padangusthasana A	[soup-TAH pod-ang-goosh-TAHS-anna]	11, **61**
Supta Padangusthasana B	[soup-TAH pod-ang-goosh-TAHS-anna]	8, **48**
Supta Padangusthasana, Bent-Knee Version	[soup-TAH pod-ang-goosh-TAHS-anna]	**54**, 76
Supta Padangusthasana, Revolving Version	[soup-TAH pod-ang-goosh-TAHS-anna]	**66**
Tadasana	[tah-DAS-anna]	106
Triang Mukhaikapada Paschimottanasana	[tree-AWN-guh moo-KA-eh-ka-paw-duh POSH-ee-moh-tun-AWS-anna]	8,9,15,**128**,136,140
Trikonasana	[trik-cone-AHS-anna]	50
Ubhaya Padangusthasana	[oub-HA-ya pod-awng-goosh-TAWS-anna]	**160**
Upavistha Konasana	[oo-pah-VEESH-tah cone-AHS-anna]	7,28,**40**,76
Uttanasana	[OOT-tan-AHS-ahna]	124

Other Sanskrit Terms	Pronunciation	Pages
Asana	[AHS-anna]	——
Ashtanga	[UHSSH-TAWN-gah]	——
Bandha	[bahn-dah]	**15**, 66, 80, 96, 120, 150
Chakra	[CHUHK-ruh]	——
Drishti	[dr-ISH-tee]	——
Hatha	[huh-tuh]	6, 12, 26
Jalandhara Bandha	[jah-lahn-DHA-rah bahn-dah]	17
Kriya	[kr-EE-yah]	——
Mudra	[MOO-drah]	——
Mula Bandha	[moo-lah bahn-dah]	15-17
Namasté	[nah-moss-te (te rhymes with day)]	——
Pranayama	[PRAH-nah-yama]	——
Udyana Bandha	[oo-dee-YAH-nah BAHN-dah]	17
Ujjayi	[oo-jy (jy rhymes with pie)-ee]	——
Vinyasa	[vin-YAH-sah]	——
Yoga	[YO-gah]	——

ENGLISH POSE INDEX

CONTRIBUTORS

CHRIS MACIVOR—a self-taught computer expert and digital artist—is the Technical Director for Bandha Yoga and Illustrator of the bestselling series, *The Key Muscles of Yoga* and *The Key Poses of Yoga*. He is a graduate of Etobicoke School of the Arts, Sheridan College, and Seneca College. With a background in dance and traditional art, as well as computer graphics and animation, Chris considers himself to be equally artistic and technical in nature. Working with Dr. Long on the Scientific Keys book series, he has digitally reproduced the biomechanical perfection of the human body. With a keen eye for subtle lighting and a passion for excellence in his art, Chris successfully brings his imagery to life.

KURT LONG, BFA, is an award-winning fine artist and anatomical illustrator who contributed the front and back cover illustrations. He is a graduate of the University of Pennsylvania and has studied at the Pennsylvania Academy of Fine Arts and the Art Students League of New York. Kurt resides in Philadelphia with his wife and two sons. For information on commissions and to see more of his work, go to www.KurtLong.net.

STEWART THOMAS contributed the Sanskrit calligraphy and the special hand-painted border for the Bandha Yoga Codex. He is an award-winning artist, calligrapher, printmaker and designer. A graduate of Haverford College and the University of the Arts in Philadelphia, he serves as Creative Director of Florida's Eden, a regional alliance working for a sustainable future for North Florida, and produces art at his own Palmstone Studio (www.palmstone.com).

ERYN KIRKWOOD, MA, RYT 200, graduated from Carleton University with a Master's Degree in English Literature. She left a corporate career as Managing Editor at the Canadian Medical Association to dedicate her life to the study, practice, and teaching of yoga. Eryn is the Chief Editor at Bandha Yoga and maintains an award-winning Blog. She offers alignment-focused yoga classes in Ottawa, Canada, and can be reached at www.BarrhavenYoga.com.

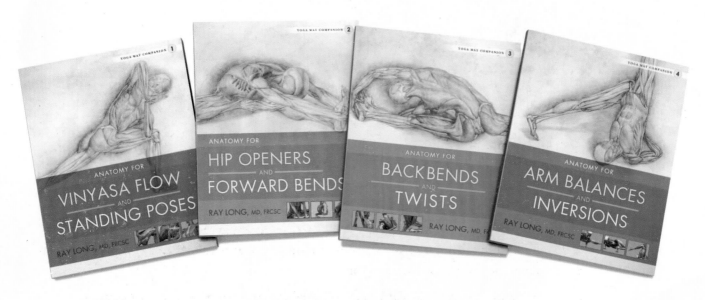

ALSO FROM BANDHA YOGA

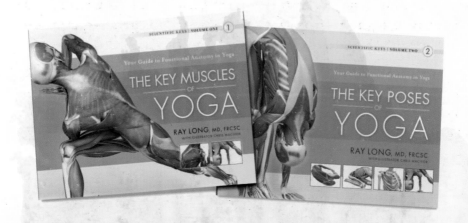

www.BandhaYoga.com